The Healing of the 1lb Baby

Marie Delanote

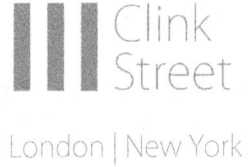

London | New York

Published by Clink Street Publishing 2014

Copyright © Marie Delanote 2014

First edition.

The author asserts the moral right under the Copyright, Designs and Patents Act 1988 to be identified as the author of this work.

All rights reserved. No part of this publication may be reproduced, stored in a retrieval system or transmitted, in any form or by any means without the prior consent of the author, nor be otherwise circulated in any form of binding or cover other than that which it is published and without a similar condition being imposed on the subsequent purchaser.

ISBN: 978-1-909477-38-4
Ebook: 978-1-909477-39-1

Contents

Introduction

PART 1: Pre-pregnancy

Chapter 1: Pre-pregnancy; written in the cards

Chapter 2: Pregnant

Chapter 3: A woman DOES know her body better than anyone else

Chapter 4: Three scary days in the unknown

Chapter 5: Transfer

Chapter 6: Energetically explained reasons for premature birth and pregnancy problems

PART 2: A new life begins; Elouisa is born

Chapter 7: Born at twenty-four weeks' pregnancy

Chapter 8: Baby development facts; 23–25 weeks' gestation

Chapter 9: Life in turmoil

Chapter 10: Psychic surgery, closing of the duct

Chapter 11: Loneliness–oneness

Chapter 12: Baby development facts; 26–28 weeks' gestation

Chapter 13: The healing of the energy-sucking new nurse
Chapter 14: Psychic surgery, go away bug
Chapter 15: Guilt towards the other children
Chapter 16: The spiritual healing doctor
Chapter 17: Adjustment to the outside world
Chapter 18: Baby development facts; 28–30 weeks' gestation
Chapter 19: Not just for me; healing of a full term baby with life threatening lung problems
Chapter 20: A baby on the ward passes away
Chapter 21: Swollen tummy and water retention
Chapter 22: Baby development facts; 31–33 weeks' gestation
Chapter 23: Eyes and ears
Chapter 24: Transfer closer to home

PART 3: Home
Chapter 25: Physical and Ethereal Crystal healing
Chapter 26: Eating

Thank you

I would like to thank all doctors, nurses, midwives, paramedics, specialists, physiologists, occupational therapists, ophthalmologist, neonatologist, audiologist, dietician, community nurses, health visitors, paediatrician, nursery ladies, the boys' teachers... who stood by our daughters, sons, me and my husband during the first two years of our Elouisa's life. The support has been incredible and beyond expectations!

I would like to thank Dorothy and Norman for their presence whenever my husband needed them during Elouisa's hospital stay and after. And a big thank you to Dot, who helped me to correct the spelling in my writing process as English is not my mother tongue. She was a major help in my achieving a presentable manuscript to submit to the publisher.

Thank you to my sister, Emmanuelle, for being there for me every step of the way during the hospital stage.

Thank you to my friends Karen and Priske, who stood by me with love and attention.

The Healing of the 1lb Baby

For answers to questions, spiritual help, healing sessions or courses, don't hesitate to contact me via mail: mariedelanote@hotmail.com

To be published next: *Heal By Intention – Crystal Learning and Oracle Cards*

Love and Light to the world,
Marie

Introduction

Every living being is perfect and full of healing power.

This book discusses the magical cooperation between medical and spiritual healing. It tells the personal journey, full of fascinating spiritual experiences and happenings that took place when my daughter was born after exactly twenty-four weeks of pregnancy weighing just one pound/535 grams.

The book uncovers what happens in the mind of the mother to 'create' the illness in the body that causes so very early a birth. How the positive thinking of the mind and realization of perfect health helped to heal our baby and have her be a perfectly healthy, normally developed child against all odds.

The book talks about psychic surgery, Universal energy healing, Crystal and Ethereal Crystal healing, family circle healing, loneliness–oneness, dark energy healing, hope and trust.

After a long and difficult awareness process, I finally started seeing 'the Light' when my fourth child was born at only 24 weeks + 1 day of pregnancy. The love towards your child is the deepest you can ever feel. The trauma that presented itself to me at that time made me realize that I am a healer, that I can do this with the help of the Universe. This was my lesson; the end of not believing in myself, of putting myself down. It was now time to stop believing what everybody had always told me while I was growing up, that all that imaginary 'stuff' is not real. Well, I am telling you, it does work and it is very real!

Our younger daughter is seen as a 'medical miracle', happy, healthy and absolutely perfect. I haven't stopped using the method of healing by intention with Ethereal Crystals, physical crystals and psychic surgery since she was born. In my practice, I make people aware of how strong our minds are, how we can heal ourselves using this method. I heal: clients, my own children, places I go to, situations in the news, stories people tell me, dogs I run into in the park... every day as I go through life. What a beautiful magical world is out there, and all I want to do is spread the word so more people use these techniques and become more aware of our powerful, healthy, happy and loving nature and the power of the unlimited Universe, which can be tapped into whenever needed if we become more mindful.

This story doesn't just give statistics, numbers and figures about premature birth and pregnancy problems; mainly it provides hope, inspiration and insights into how and why.

The book is not just for parents of premature babies. It is a spiritual revelation and interesting to any person, worldwide. It is a genuine, inspirational, true story.

Part 1: Pre-pregnancy

Chapter 1: Pre-pregnancy; written in the cards

When there is a strong desire to have a baby most of us think, 'Fabulous, let's count to the fertile days, have sex, become pregnant, enjoy a relaxed pregnancy, baby kicking in the tummy, eating all the desired goodies, shopping for the little one, push the baby out without epidural because it can't be that painful, and then mooch around in total happiness with a newborn baby'.

Indeed, I was one of those people who thought this.

With my first, a boy, it was like that until after the delivery. An epidural was needed, but I could live with that. Overwhelmed by unforeseen pain I had no problem at all with having that big needle stuck into my back. I ended up with piles after giving birth. That was the result of the forced pushing whenever I was told to push; it was all too unnatural and no one had listened to my body. It was my first child. I didn't have a clue and listened to the medical staff like a good girl.

My first son, Jack, was a very demanding baby, keeping

me busy day and night. How I eventually got to four children? That is still the question. Now, nine years later he is still a very strong character but has a very kind nature. I love him to bits, but he is a handful to bring up.

Jack has lived many lives before, he is an old soul and has shared several lives with me. We have/had a lot of karma to solve. Beside his spirit guides and Guardian Angels, he has a big brown bear standing next to him. Enough said!

Before having Jack, I was still at university, living in Antwerp, a big city, with lots of friends around me. After he was born, we moved to the French-speaking area of the country. I felt very lonely and had no friends or family around; the pink cloud very quickly turned into a grey one. My husband didn't understand what was going on and felt I was just being a stroppy, annoying, difficult woman. In truth, I felt very tired, misunderstood and completely alone.

I was breastfeeding and it drove me completely bonkers! I was a hundred per cent behind the decision to breastfeed. It is so healthy, easy and the best. But in combination with feeling so tired, down on myself and uncomfortable in my own skin, having this demanding child constantly wanting to suck me empty, no matter how great the love for him, made me feel angry, and then feelings of guilt for feeling angry would take over. It became a very uncomfortable circle.

I missed the understanding and support from outside, someone who would tell me that there was nothing wrong with me.

I am sure that many other women have felt/feel this way. If you do, I strongly advise you to talk about it, and if the person you're telling doesn't understand how you feel, talk to someone else and get help in whatever way works for you! Having a baby can be terribly tiring up to the point of losing yourself.

Despite feeling the way I did, the longing for another baby

was strong. I knew that another boy was waiting to come.

I wanted Jack to stop breastfeeding and take the bottle so I could have another baby. Breastfeeding partly protects against another pregnancy and also I just knew I didn't want one in the tummy and one on the breast.

One day I sat down and told Jack firmly that there was no choice. He had to drink that bottle. At that moment a little boy with big blue eyes 'appeared' on my right side about 50 cm higher than me. I had a vision. He was 'telling' Jack to get on with it because he wanted to come. He gave out a feeling of slight irritation – 'Come on, Jack'.

Straight after that beautiful appearance, Jack drank his bottle of milk and I knew a blue eyed, bossy boy was coming our way. Two months later, I found out I was pregnant. The way I saw and felt him at that time is just the way he talks to Jack now, if, in his opinion, Jack is not quick enough.

Again my pregnancy went smoothly. Physically there were no problems but mentally and emotionally I was treading the same path as before. Lonely, misunderstood, absolutely shattered and bored senseless, which didn't help my morale. I even remember telling my sister of being very worried about slipping into a depression once the baby was born.

I had graduated at the Royal College of Music as a double bassist but once Jack was born it was a natural decision to no longer pursue my work so I could look after him, and any future children, seeing that my husband had a full time job. I was fine with that but now actually felt completely useless, as if I lost my identity. Andy didn't understand how unsatisfied I was but, in the meantime, what could he do?... No matter how often I told myself how important it was I was there for my children, I didn't feel like I was someone; this was not how I had envisaged a happy life.

When my second boy was ready to come I was convinced I

wanted to keep control during labour – it was my body and I was the only one who knew what I felt. This time I went to a hospital in France, just over the border from where we lived.

Arriving at the hospital, I was put on a monitor for forty-five minutes, on my back! I couldn't go anywhere because I was stuck on a machine, completely unable to 'catch' the contractions. Not one nurse or midwife gave any advice or had any sympathy and, again, even though it was another hospital, even another country, everything had to run on the same lines: a woman must give birth, flat on her back on a table!

Adam was a 'star watcher', he was looking chin up when he was ready to come out. The doctor first had to twist his head so he could come out. Once he was born I asked Andy to take him, I was exhausted and just wanted to be left alone to sleep. A second depression had arrived.

My lovely boy Adam has energy which is light, gentle and fairy-like. It is his second time on Earth; he brings light around him and makes people happy, but, as I saw when he appeared to Jack and I, he is very bossy and likes structure and control; he likes everything to be perfect.

Throughout my life I can remember seeing 'people' at night. I was intrigued by Oracle cards, palmistry and especially witchcraft. I regularly visited a lady who would read my cards or read and heal my chakras and aura. Ann, she was called. She would pick me up again, every time, and push me forward in the knowledge that I am a happy, important person like everybody else. Through the years I would follow courses here and there – numerology, reiki, which would give me a boost every time. It is such a fascinating world.

Ann was like a mother to me. I met her when I was nineteen. Every time I was there, she would speak the right words; she pushed me forward every time I went on a downward spiral. A good deal of healing on family bonds, past lives, my energy system was carried out. I felt as though a veil were being lifted layer by layer.

One day when Jack and Adam were still little I asked her if I could learn what she did. She said that anyone can do it but you have to be ready and be on a certain awareness level. She agreed to teach me and a new, fascinating world opened up.

In October Andy and I got married. It was a surprisingly quickly arranged wedding. Many people organize for a whole year beforehand for a perfect nuptial. For some reason, which became clear later, we decided to get married and organized everything in about four weeks. Family and friends came over from England, we had a lovely meal, they stayed over in gîtes and the wedding day itself was fantastic. The restaurant was brilliant, the weather was fabulous, we couldn't have asked for a better day.

My life was full of ups and downs with mood swings, depressive feelings, up one minute, down the next, difficult days, good days… but I kept going. To me it was, even though not always pleasant, normal.

In my heart I knew spiritual activities were an essential part of my being and it was this that would make me feel 'alive', but it simply wasn't happening. However, a series of events crossed my path and I would realize later there was a good deal of learning to be done.

For the day after the wedding we had organized a private bus to take guests back to England. My brother in law, Stuart, Andy's younger brother, gave me a big goodbye hug. He was a lovely man and worked with young teenagers from difficult backgrounds in Hackney, London. He was taller then Andy, very skinny with wild black curly hair, friendly eyes and an enormous smile – his trademark! He said, 'So lovely to see you again, the boys are a credit to you and Andy, see you soon, yeah' and waved. As he ran back to the bus I had a vision, I saw how he would die very soon.

I was so shocked and waved it away, feeling angry with my 'weird head'.

Exactly three months later, my husband called me from his office. Stuart had been taken ill and was in hospital in Spain. Andy was called to visit him. Was it serious? We didn't know, it was like a whirlwind, weird, unreal.

A few hours later I drove into town with the boys. I decided to send out (mentally) Universal energy to Stuart. Even though I had learned a good deal by this time, I still doubted my ability. However, I did it anyway and shortly after, Stuart 'came to me' and said, 'Thank you, but don't, it is my time to go'.

I felt shocked by the experience and again thought it was my imagination working overtime. An hour later my husband called me with the news that Stuart had crossed over. He passed away at forty-one years of age, an incredible person and loved by all who knew him.

The next few months passed in a daze. Andy was away for ages and I felt, again, left on my own. While everyone was trying to come to terms with Stuart's death, I had no one to talk to. I felt as if I were not allowed to say how I felt about the whole situation.

As a result my mood spiralled downwards. I had days of low energy and spirit. I even toyed with the thought of leaving everything behind and going away. I wanted to pack my bags and go; the feeling of being completely drained played heavily. This showed me how tired and depressed I had become. I could never leave my children, they are my everything – I don't even leave them with a babysitter! My mind couldn't handle it any more and Andy didn't have a clue. I lay in bed and didn't want to get up; I felt I could no longer handle the constant demands expected of me. Lying there, I became aware I needed help – it was a small amount of sanity that made me get up and go to Andy, where I collapsed and cried. A decision was made to see our doctor, who confirmed depression and prescribed anti-depressants. Normally they take a few weeks to 'kick in', but the fact that my husband knew, the doctor had listened and I was understood meant that within a few days I felt better. A small ray of hope was stealing through the darkness.

Day by day, the feeling of being stronger and more relaxed in my head increased. My husband understood me a little more and knew he had to help me out and take over when everything became too much to handle alone.

Now I gradually began to notice that these 'down' periods would last three weeks and then there was a week's break...

As the months went by and I began to feel stronger, out of the blue I was asked to teach Dutch to French speaking children at a local school. I knew this wasn't what I fully wanted to do, but I took the opportunity and loved it. Earning money of my own gave me independence and boosted my confidence and morale. People knew me and I finally felt fully accepted in the small community I lived in.

Slowly but surely the longing for another child crept in. I knew a little girl was waiting in the wings; the desire for a daughter became very strong. My husband became worried I would fall back into the same mood traps. I knew if another pregnancy were to happen I should stop taking the anti-depressants as they would not be good for the baby.

An acupuncturist helped me to gently let go of the medication.

I fell pregnant again, immediately. The test said 'no' but I knew 'yes', so went to see a doctor for confirmation. He did a blood test. Several waiting days followed before receiving the results. My whole body was showing signs of pregnancy so these few days were a terribly long wait. When finally the saving phone call came I was excitedly running up the stairs to tell Andy while listening to the doctor. Andy and the boys were decorating the boys' bedroom. As I came to the top of the stairs and the doctor told me I was pregnant but it was still very early days so he would want to take another blood test a week later, another vision came. On my right side about 50 cm above my head level, my brother-in-law Stuart, who was smiling broadly, in full glory looked at me; on his right side sat a young girl, about ten years old, with long hair, also smiling at me. The feeling that this was my daughter completed the whole picture. These visions happen in a split second but are so clear. It was a beautiful vision and I knew Stuart was safe and happy. Andy and I had decided we didn't want to know the sex of the baby we were having, but, of course I already knew.

I kept up my weekly sessions with the acupuncturist, which reduced the morning sickness and kept my morale high. The whole nine months felt fabulous.

A flyer came through the door about how to prepare for a successful birth. The lady who offered this service had been a midwife at the local hospital, which I felt comfortable with. It was thanks to her that the hope for an enjoyable birth became real. These helpful lessons, which included breathing exercises and short meditation, felt good.

On the first of September the whole process began. As we drove to the hospital, mixed emotions of happiness and sadness flowed through me. I had always enjoyed being pregnant but felt sad that this would be the last time. Tears rolled down my cheeks. My husband, Andy, didn't really want more than two children so with an expected daughter on the way I felt my luck was being pushed to the limit.

Because I was now in a different hospital from the last pregnancies I was fortunate that my gynaecologist there was fabulous. She was so sensitive and in connection with my situation. Thanks to the exercises during my pregnancy and the acupuncture, I felt in full control. There was no lying on tables or being told what to do. I was guided and relaxed and allowed my body to tell me what to do, every step of the way. The gynaecologist called me 'Chief'. The waters stayed intact until the minute the baby came out. The big moment then was to see what we had, and, as I well knew, even though Andy called out 'It's another boy', it was, of course, a girl. And this time, after two grey clouds, I was floating on a pinky cloud nine.

With the help of acupuncture, chakra healing and better sleep, I fully enjoyed my third child.

The healing of guilt feelings towards my boys, because I didn't feel good after their births, is another story and, luckily, has now taken place.

Chakras are energy – our consciousness centres in and outside our body. We cannot physically detect our chakras, they are energy connections to our aura (the energy field around us) and the energy world around us.

Chakra means 'turning wheel of light'.

Chakras have a direct influence on the organs, blood stream, organ functions, hormones, emotions and thoughts! Also, the other way around, the mind has a direct influence on the chakras. It is crucially important that we keep the energy flowing evenly through the whole body so that life is physically, mentally and emotionally lived in balance.

Many of us have lived many times before. Every emotional, physical, psychological happening through all these lives has been stored in the energy system, in the chakras.

So the physical body and mind is the result of the energetic system.

We need to clear away the negative hang-ups of the past so that we can live in light, love and happiness – our natural state. People think we need to 'suffer' to grow, but we grow even more when we live a happy life.

Every chakra is in connection with a specific physical and psychological function. Negative psychological and emotional feelings eventually cause disharmony in our energy system.

A disharmonized energy system changes how we view life, how we think and feel and it stops us from living a full and happy life. The joy of life will fade and the conscious level will drop; eventually this will lead to disease and pain.

Heal your chakras, happenings, emotions and mind, and

feel, think and live happily!!! The chakras are explained further in my book *Heal by Intention – Crystal Learning and Oracle Cards*.

The one chakra that is crucially important here, in this story, is the Sacral chakra, the chakra that causes pregnancy problems and premature birth if blocked.

The Sacral chakra, second chakra, has its place inside the body, 2 cm below the belly button. It is not physically detectable; it is a wheel of energy.

A healthy Sacral chakra creates:
- Sexuality
- Propagation
- Creativity
- Self consciousness
- Emotions
- Sense: Taste
- The right to feel
- Colour: Orange

A blocked Sacral chakra creates:
- Guilt

Addictions linked to the Sacral chakra:
- Sex
- Alcohol
- Heroin

Our Sacral chakra can get blocked by the following events:
- Inherited traumas of parents around sexuality
- Rejection
- Alcoholic families
- Religious or moral severity against lust
- Sexual and physical abuse
- Emotional violence
- Emotional manipulation
- Any situation linked to emotional stress

- Personality severaly stifled by parents
- Unstable situation
- Neglect

Physical problems that can occur caused by a blockage of this chakra:
- Mood swings
- Periods staying away/menstruation problems
- Prostate problems
- Problems with the male sexual organ
- Cancer of uterus and ovaries
- Early menopause
- Fertility problems
- Middle back pain
- Disorders: Semen, urine, blood, lymph
- Premature delivery
- PMS
- Postnatal depression
- Obesity
- Infections
- Preeclampsia
- Disorders of the uterus and ovaries

The three weeks down and one week up emotions I had experienced now became clear. I had suffered severe PMS for a very long time. This, together with postnatal depression after the birth of my two boys, had added to my problem. Nobody ever mentioned PMS, I had to discover this by myself while reading books and the internet and following spiritual courses.

When I analyse myself, I finally understand why I felt the way I did, why I had PMS, moods swings and postnatal depression.

Through readings I found out I had had many lives of emotional manipulation and suppression. I was, always, in different ways, not allowed to be whom I was. On top of that, I was carrying current family circle energies. On my father's side there was religious severity against lust and emotional manipulation. Signs of excessive alcohol use started to show in the family.

On my mother's side guilt and shame were carried through heavily. As far back as I can go it became seriously stuck in the relationship between my great grandmother and my grandfather, who had fostered a love–hate relationship and feelings of rejection. This is the whole thing with family circle energies, parents (unconsciously!) pass them on to their children.

Added to my energy being burdened with this past, I suffered a huge amount of stress as a young child when my parents went through a divorce. The relationship with my first stepmother was nothing like an enjoyable one, which made the stress levels and emotions run high from the age of five.

It is very clear to me that all of these happenings caused a blockage to my Sacral chakra, the centre of emotions, sexuality and creativity.

Because my Sacral chakra became blocked, the results in my case were PMS, severe mood swings and postnatal depression. The thing was that, except for Andy (partly), no one knew how I felt. It happened deep inside, like a beast that wasn't allowed to come out. The outside world knew me as a happy, smiley young woman with not a thing to worry about; I just got on with it; this is how life was for me. What could I do? It was only after my fourth child was born that I learned to heal deeply; pull out the roots and keep up 'the maintenance'. Heal the body; heal the mind. Heal the mind; heal the body. Heal the chakras; heal the body and mind. Throw off the heavy coat of past burdens and live life in a natural state of perfect health, whole love and full happiness.

I finally saw that family circles also had to be healed to 'free' my own children. This is how we move towards a happier life and planet. Pull out the roots of past lives and family circles, heal your chakras to stop encroaching further into the family and live in your natural state.

I had found a very good 'Lenormand' Oracle card reader via a nursery lady. Full of enthusiasm, I had to go and see her. She was brilliant. Not everyone would like the Lenormand cards seeing that they are very confrontational and straightforward – they see actual life happenings.

I had felt for a while, after my daughter was born, that a girl and a boy both wanted to come to our family, but it became clear that the next pregnancy wouldn't go well, perhaps not even result in a baby at all. The one after would be fine.

One of the things Clara, the card reader, mentioned was that she saw big health problems with a child. I panicked straight away, thinking of my three children. She saw very big problems, she was worried herself and I remember her saying how she really didn't like seeing this. There would be hospitals involved, but at the end, no one would die, at the end all looked fine. She first said I would get pregnant but would miscarry. Two minutes later she said in full confusion, 'Oh, you will have a baby anyway'. When she told me about the miscarriage I felt this would not be so.

This part of the reading was still a bit of a mystery so I let it go.

My husband, Andy, is always ready for new adventures. He will have an idea and the world will have to move. In September 2011 it happened again. We were living in Belgium when he came up with the idea to move to the UK, his home country. It had to happen straight away. Our son Jack had just started primary school so he wouldn't lose too much of the school year. Four weeks later, we were in England.

At the point we decided to make the move Andy was just leaving to cycle from Spain to the UK for the charity he had set up in honour of his brother Stuart. So once again, it was up to me to sort everything out. He left, and I had to arrange the move, on my own and only in four weeks, not forgetting I was still teaching part time.

I still don't think he realized what a big thing this was for me. He was coming back to where he grew up. For me, it was a new country, a new language and they were driving on the other side of the road, which I had never done before!

On top of that, nursery schools in the UK are very expensive, so while the boys could go to school, my one year old daughter would have to stay at home until the age of five. In Belgium, I had fought myself out of loneliness, got a job, met new people and brought the kids to school and nursery.

Now I would be back to square one, no job, no nursery and no friends. This is what I thought.

I grabbed life with both hands, though, refusing to go down. I loved the place we moved to: An old psychiatric institution, beautifully renovated. I had felt 'all sorts' the second I arrived but it also felt good. Very often I felt watched but it didn't feel uncomfortable.

I had been sixteen years old when I'd first met Paul, an astrologist and card reader. He was thirty years older than me when I first visited his spiritual shop to have my cards read. He also taught me the basics of numerology. I had always felt comfortable with him, he was kind and caring like a father figure. I hadn't seen him again after my move to the south of Belgium, just before Jack was born. At the end of October 2010 , he called me out of the blue, to see if he could come and stay in our B&B with his partner. We had opened a three-bedroom B&B to create an extra income and in the future, making it easier to sell the house.

I was so happy and felt valued in our 'relationship'.

When he arrived, another vision appeared. Again, it happened in less then a second; it was a knowing. 'He looks ill, he is going to pass away.'

I tried to push away this thought, seeing that he was acting fine and happy.

They booked in for two nights but only stayed one. His mother in law suddenly became ill and needed them. Apparently this always happened when they were away on a trip.

It felt like a flying trip. He arrived, and before I knew it, he was gone.

Two months later, just before the big England move, I was desperate to learn to read the Oracle cards 'Lenormand'. I thought it would make sense to learn them in my own language, so tried to contact Paul again, to see if he could help me with this study. There was no answer so I checked up on the 'net. I found out he had passed away. That last visit was his goodbye and my vision had come true.

This was in September 2011. I remember sitting at my computer with my arms open reaching up high praying to Paul to help me find someone who would teach me to read the 'Lenormand' cards. Anxiety and a slight fear took over because I didn't want to find a charlatan. By 'coincidence' Toni's name seemed to attract my attention, so I checked out what was going on around him. The other problem was that I would have to find someone who would drive for two hours or more to come to my house. I was living in the French-speaking part of the country whilst searching for a Flemish-speaking card reader. And on top of that, Andy was away, so coping with three children on my own meant that the teacher would have to come to me. Toni's name kept popping up and it felt good so I gave him a ring, offering him a free weekend with his wife in our B&B, stating I would pay him for card reading lessons. When he accepted the offer I couldn't believe my luck!

Thank you, Paul, for helping!

When Toni and his wife arrived it became clear that he'd known Paul very well. There you go, how beautifully does the Universe work!

Toni didn't come in with just the Lenormand cards, he also brought a course in the cards 'Belline', 'Tarot' and palmistry. He taught me all weekend. It was perfect. He came the weekend my in-laws were there to look after the children so the lessons proceeded even better than I could have imagined.

One of the things Toni mentioned when he read my hands was that I would have a miscarriage next time I was pregnant. He couldn't see this pregnancy working out well.

Of course it is impossible to completely understand three different types of Oracle cards and palmistry in just two days, but thanks to written courses, I could keep studying and practising after he left. He looked in my hands and told me to never give up, that when he saw me in ten years' time, he wanted me to have succeeded and be thriving. 'With such spiritual hands, I am jealous,' he said. 'You are on the right path, keep going!' This whole experience was a 'butt kick' from above, a new lesson to show me my path. Even though deep inside I have always felt the happiest being busy with those practices, the doubts in myself and this path were always there.

So, we ended up in England!

Every time my daughter went for a nap, I sat at my little desk practising and learning the cards.

Then it was time for another awakening. My father visited me in England, bringing along two friends, and that's how I met a now very dear friend, Carine.

I walked to greet them outside the building (the ex-psychiatric institution). When I saw Carine, she constantly had a puzzled expression on her face. It seemed weird that she was there. We didn't know her or her husband and they seemed a little uncomfortable. I hadn't seen my dad in a while and Carine and her husband felt they shouldn't be there. I discovered shortly afterwards that whenever

Carine had tried to put a stop to their visit something had happened which led her towards England, accompanying Dad and his partner.

Once we were in the house, my dad's partner took out the Lenormand cards that I had asked her to bring and then everything fell into place. Carine sighed loudly and said, 'Now I understand! I am into healing and "they" (spirit guides and Angels) brought me here, because I needed to tell you that you should bring these earthbound spirits in this building to the Light!' That was it, we chatted and didn't stop. Wow, impressive. 'They' had drawn Carine to my house to tell me this. I had been ignoring these spirits, who were stuck in the psychiatric institution, thinking I was imagining them, so Carine was sent to stop me ignoring them and start healing. So this was also why we ended up living in that building. Carine mentioned that once the job was done, we would move and that would be in about two months' time. Indeed, this is what did happen.

Earthbound spirits are people who died but never went to the Light. It scared them, so they stayed where they had passed away. Clearly the people who lived in the psychiatric institution had had a very hard life.

It was an experience out of this world. I had never done anything like this before and it was mind blowing. Luckily Carine warned me that some of them didn't realize they were dead, so I would have to protect myself and be persistent.

Indeed, during one of the healing days, it was suddenly like a wind being displaced from twenty metres away to right in front of me. A fearsome man stood very close and looked me straight in the eyes. It felt that he was keeping everyone (the earthbound spirits) in check, as if he was in charge in their world. I told him 'You are dead, go to the Light'. My heart was pounding but I just kept telling him he was dead and he had to go to the Light and waved my hand from him to the Light until I felt the energy softening and he went up into the sky to the light I had called for. I was buzzing for the rest of the day. What an experience.

Even though I hadn't felt sadness in the building, once the healing commenced, big groups (especially of women) were clinging onto each other, full of fear. It was a relief seeing them go to the Light, to the place where they should be and where they would be looked after.

This work spread over a period of about fifteen days. Even when we were just walking around the building things occurred. For example, in a little building within the confines of the complex, it came through to me that hundreds of babies had died there in the past due to illegally performed abortions. Their spirits had become 'stuck' and thanks to an opening Light above the building I was able to release them.

From then onwards the spirits sought me out. They were clearly ready to go to the Light. They were mostly single spirits who found me even when I was showering. They always seemed to appear when I was alone, when the work could be done straight away. Even spirits not belonging to the building showed up. Once, I was sitting in my car when a young man appeared. He made it clear (in my mind, with a picture and a knowing) that he had passed away in a car accident but couldn't go to the Light because his family were grieving so badly, they wouldn't let him go. I then followed my intuition, 'cut' him loose from his family, put reiki healing symbols in place and helped him to the Light.

Chapter 2: Pregnant

Several times before, I had had the feeling that there were a girl and boy still 'sitting' with me. Already, months before, I had told a friend that, if I were to have another baby, something wouldn't be right. Another child would come, but the next pregnancy wouldn't flow like the others. The feeling that I might even end up with no baby was there as well. But it was certain that I would have another child. Now, that was also hard to believe seeing that Andy did not want any more. We had gone through deep financial problems and climbed out again. We both knew that I needed to do something for myself, which wasn't possible until the children were of school age, that being from five years old in England. If we were to have another child, it would mean staying at home for another five years and I knew I couldn't do that. It feels so good now being able to say this without guilt. It doesn't make me a bad mother because I like being me within and having my own potential and personal life goals. This is not selfish and has absolutely nothing to do with the love I feel towards my children.

At the end of January I was a week late with my period. That doesn't happen to me as I am usually on the dot and never late, except when pregnant. I was on the phone talking with one of my sisters when she said in demanding voice, 'For goodness' sake Marie, go into the toilet and wee on that stick!' I don't know why I had been ignoring this; scared to find out I suppose.

And yes, I was pregnant! This was not planned. I had stopped the birth control pill after having Orla-Jane, my daughter, because all those hormones did not help the PMS at all and only made it worse. After stopping the pill, the PMS had reduced massively. We both now knew in our hearts that IF another child came we would be over the moon. Our life was reorganized, there were no problems and on top of that I knew exactly when it was 'fertile time' so the husband had to keep away. Well, what happened, I don't know, but clearly something changed the cycle because, yes, I was pregnant.

I didn't say anything to my husband and just left the test on the table for when he came home. I can tell you, I have never seen him lost for words; it was actually very funny. He was absolutely speechless. So, lesson one, you don't always know when you can get pregnant!

Andy panicked straight away, with half a smile on his face. Happy, confused, nervous. We were renting a three bedroom apartment – we had to move! So the world had to move again.. Five weeks later, we were living in a comfortable, spacious four bedroom house.

With the other children I had felt fully pregnant straight away, telling everyone who wanted to hear it. This time I kept it quiet. The gut feeling was, what if something went wrong? I remembered what Clara and Toni had said and also my own instinct about the potential coming pregnancy.

When living in Belgium, a pregnant woman is followed up by a gynaecologist monthly. Every month a scan is made to check the development, growth and health of the baby. On top of that, blood and urine tests are made to check for toxoplasmosis, CMV, Streptococcus B and the protein level in the urine.

Here is a short explanation of these bacteria to help you understand why this testing is done.

Toxoplasmosis:
Toxoplasmosis is caused by a very small parasite (*Toxoplasma gondii*) that infects cats particularly, but via the eggs in the stool it can infect other animals too.

Infection happens via cat stools, infected water, soil, sand, unwashed veg and fruit and (not sufficiently heated) meat. If infected before being pregnant, a woman will build up immunity, and a blood test can confirm whether this has happened. If infected during pregnancy there are few or no symptoms in the woman. The unborn child can develop problems linked to the nervous system or eye diseases or the woman will miscarry.

If you are infected while you're pregnant, treatment is available. Treatment can reduce the risk of the baby becoming infected. Where the baby is infected, treatment may reduce the risk of damage.

CMV:
Cytomegalovirus is a virus transmitted via urine and saliva particularly of children between one and four years old. The virus nests in the body fluids: urine, saliva, stools, mother's milk, blood, tears, sperm and vaginal fluid. If the unborn child is affected, it can develop severe brain and eye damage. The child can also get infected during birth.

CMV is a common virus that is part of the herpes family of viruses. It causes few symptoms in most people. If you do experience symptoms, they may be similar to flu or glandular fever and include a high temperature (fever), a sore throat and swollen glands.

Streptococcus B:
Streptococcus B is a bacterium. Pregnant women sometimes carry this bacterium in the vagina. In most cases this does not cause any problems, but it can make a small number of babies very ill if they are infected by this bacterium. In general, Streptococcus B can be treated with antibiotics. Sometimes this bacterium will cause bladder infection, which is then detectable in a culture of the urine.

About half of women that carry strep B give this to their child during labour. If one in five pregnant women carry this, ten per cent of all newborn babies will be infected. Not all babies become ill, most of the time the bacterium stays on the skin or mucosa of the baby. Babies only get ill if the bacterium penetrates the body. This happens in one in a thousand newborns.

If the mother carries strep B, the bacterium becomes an infection and the fluid-filled membranes (amniotic sac) are damaged, the baby can get infected. The bacterium goes from the vagina into the uterus, where it infects the amniotic fluids. The baby swallows the amniotic and it is taken into the lungs. If not treated quickly, it can be fatal for the baby.

These are all infection types that have the potential to cause devastation for an unborn baby. Interestingly, a link can be made to what was mentioned earlier in Chapter one. Infection is one of the physical appearances of the Sacral chakra being blocked. The mind, because of certain experiences in past and/or present lives, cannot take any more/needs a break, so creates physical problems. When the emotional stress level becomes too high (emotions have their seat in the Sacral chakra), an infection or accident happens. If one is pregnant, this can result in the unborn baby being affected, pregnancy problems and premature delivery. It is as a protection of the mind for the self, i.e. 'I need to look after myself so need to alienate what has been added – the baby'. Don't misunderstand me, this happens at a very deep unconscious level of the mind.

All that has happened to our emotions, creativity, sexuality has made scars deep in the mind, so it wants to protect itself; or the mind is too 'scared' to reproduce itself in the way of offspring. It is a way of protecting precious babies from 'this world' that has caused you so much pain. Very deep down, the mind will create physical malformations or problems, so reproduction cannot happen; or when it does happen, it tries to stop it.

This is a process that happens in such deep unconscious levels that it cannot be taken as personal or bad or guilt-full.

The maternity system in the UK shocked me. It was very different so I had to get my head around the fact that I would only have a scan at twelve and twenty weeks during pregnancy. Blood tests that I was used to were just not happening. I had Streptococcus B when pregnant with Orla-Jane in Belgium. The gynaecologist didn't want to take any risks and when labour started, she gave me antibiotics. When Orla-Jane was born, she was also given antibiotics. As this was the case in my last pregnancy, I was very concerned that no one seemed to pay any attention to this, this time.

I booked myself in privately to have a seven week scan. I started showing and the feeling of a not good pregnancy made me very insecure.

On the day of the scan I was so nervous, almost waiting for the doctor to tell me I was not pregnant or that something wasn't right.

She told us everything was perfect, I was seven weeks pregnant and the baby was developing as it should. The excitement was enormous. Maybe I was wrong after all and all would be well. When I asked for a blood test for 'feared' diseases I could not get one unless I paid about five hundred pounds. There was nothing I could do, I would have to trust and accept that a test of this kind wasn't done here. My husband reassured me that with so many women in the UK giving birth every year, clearly the risk of getting these infections was very small, otherwise these tests would be routine. I decided to have them done in Belgium when I returned.

One lunchtime I stood in the kitchen. The children were busy around me and my husband was in the bedroom. We were still in the apartment and the master bedroom was just off the kitchen and the lounge. Andy was sitting on the bed with the laptop, booking the boys into some fun day camps for the holidays.

Another vision. A young man walked from the bedroom where Andy was sitting to where I stood. He turned around to look at Andy and then at me. He gave me the very strong feeling of saying goodbye. Next, he was gone. I just stood there. As I had always felt a boy and a girl in the wings and this just happened, I knew that a little girl was growing in my tummy.

Chapter 3: A woman DOES know her body better than anyone else

Our next move was into a lovely spacious four bedroom house. Andy was away a lot with work. Juggling with the three children and being pregnant was all becoming too much.

I found myself an acupuncturist as this had helped me so much during the last pregnancy. It helped again so the sickness wasn't too bad during the first twelve weeks.

At the time of the twelve week scan, all was chaos. One misunderstanding after another occurred. The hospital told me the scan would be done somewhere else, which I thought was the community hospital, but nobody there knew who I was. I rang another hospital but they couldn't find me on the list. I was so stressed and upset and desperately missed my friendly, helpful, Belgian gynaecologist. I rang Andy in tears. He had attended the seven week scan but had work commitments at this time so was unable to come.

I eventually arranged another appointment for a scan. The receptionist was horrible –looked at me disparagingly as if I should know how the hospital system worked in England. I was again sent from here to there, because 'don't you know that you need a urine sample before you go upstairs!' was her unfriendly and unhelpful comment. Clearly, not having gone through a pregnancy in England before, I did not. Luckily Andy came with me, which made me feel stronger, and after the scan I received extra pictures from the ultrasonographer and was assured our baby was fine.

When we told Andy's family, his mother was very excited; his father said in an emotionless voice, 'No, how did that happen?' That really upset me. As if you are stupid to have four children. Questioning us about finances seemed the last straw. It did appear as if from the beginning things did not flow as they should.

During our chat with the midwife, I was very impressed. She asked me how my mental state had been during and after pregnancy. Halleluiah! No one had ever asked me that before. She gave me the phone number of a psychologist in case I had any problems. Mental health problems were recognized in this country!

I went to Belgium for the Easter holidays and visited my gynaecologist. At this time I was sixteen weeks into my pregnancy so had a scan and blood test. I felt on top of the world and started to forget my doubts, premonitions and fears. Perhaps everyone had been wrong, myself included. I started to enjoy the pregnancy. Wow, four children, I felt so proud, this was pure wealth!

The weeks passed. Andy was away again. I felt so angry with him for 'leaving' me with 'all the work', as I saw it. It is so important to have feedback and support from a partner when you have small children. Ours were twenty months, and five and six years old. It was a hard time and I felt tired, upset, unsupported and guilty. It seemed I wasn't allowed to feel this way because I had everything to make me happy. I was placing myself in the position of a victim when I wasn't a victim, which was an old ingrown family string. I was battling between feelings of low self esteem and the knowledge that I was very worthy and fantastic. I was so scared that my other children would pick up on my moods or feel less loved that I would do everything they asked me to. I would even carry them one by one up the stairs when it was bedtime. I was now over twenty weeks pregnant! The feeling that I was unworthy of this baby grew. How would I cope? An enormous inner battle was going on here.

The strange thing was that during this pregnancy I seemed to attract negative reactions. The more I felt down on myself, the more unsympathetic people would be towards my having four children.

On one occasion a teacher at the school made blunt comments such as 'Yes, well, you wanted four children...' or 'with all your children...', always with a negative tone. It felt as if a heavy blanket was burying me in its folds and I would be down all day.

One of the mothers in school would unload her whole history of miscarriages and her sadness that she only had one child. She would look me in the eye and say, 'My daughter is sometimes sad that she doesn't have a sibling. Well, people with more children don't have the time to spend proper time with their children... how will you do this with four!'

I am incredibly sensitive, I pick up on everyone's moods and feelings, it was not funny.

There is a reason why your partner is your partner; we all learn certain lessons from each other. Andy taught me to stand up for myself if people are unfriendly, 'to kill them with kindness', not to stand in the victim position.

I just couldn't put it into practice yet. The anger from within towards him was getting so big, but I didn't say anything. I was scared of looking silly, to be the over dramatizing woman. I was scared he would have had enough and leave...

On the 5th of May 2012, when I was 21 weeks + 4 days pregnant, I woke up with pain in my throat. It felt very swollen and I had difficulty swallowing. This came as no surprise. I was aware now that the body reacts to the mind. For so long now I had felt that Andy made all the decisions and I just had to follow, so I just kept my mouth shut and let the anger fester inside me. I couldn't change it anyway. Even if I did tell him, what could he do? So it was no surprise that my throat, the energy point of communication, had become blocked. Much later it would become clear that it was an infection; infection is linked to a blockage in the chakra of emotions.

I couldn't say (Throat chakra, heart of communication, can bring pain in the throat when blocked) what I felt (Sacral chakra, heart of the emotions, can result in infection when blocked). Result, I developed an infection in the throat. The nasty beast, Streptococcus A.

Streptococcus A is a bacterium that spreads via direct contact with mucus from the nose or throat of an infected person. A strep A infection is to be found in the nose, pharynx and on the skin or in infected wounds. This type of infection can infect the kidneys, heart valves, meninges and the uterus. When worried about strep A, the doctor can take a sample from the throat to detect the bacteria and give antibiotics. This type of streptococcus is potentially fatal.

In a few hours' time my whole throat felt blocked. I couldn't drink or eat. I was swallowing pus and had intense throat pain. I was in absolute agony.

We went to do some shopping but I stayed in the car. I sat there, crying, not knowing how to sit to be comfortable.

I couldn't do anything. Thank goodness it was the weekend and Andy was home so he could take over.

It could be said that one of the children had it so I just caught it, but the explanation is that a healthy body's vibration is always higher than that of a bacterium... It is only when the energy level is down that the beast can dig its claws into you...

At that point I didn't know what I had. Andy kept comforting me, saying that it would pass. He was just trying to settle me. I was worried sick, literally. All the past predictions and visions came back. That night we should have gone out to celebrate a friend's birthday, instead I stayed at home and checked the internet. The name Streptococcus A came up and I recognized all the signs. When I kept reading what it could do when the victim is pregnant, it was like someone was ringing the bell of time... that's it, this is it.

I turned to the Oracle cards 'Belline' and asked what was going on. I picked the card '17 Disease'. Healthwise this card means infection, diseases or worse.

Again, Andy tried to comfort me by saying that I was just imagining things and that I shouldn't make any judgments based on the internet and he suggested I go to see a doctor.

The next day I made an appointment and a weekend doctor saw me, someone I did not know. I told him about my concerns and the potential strep A. (I did not tell him about the Oracle card, I thought he might send me to a mental institution!)

The doctor waved all my worries away. I asked for a blood test but he said that wasn't needed. I was just an over worried mother-to-be and I shouldn't read all these things on the internet. He advised that I did not need an antibiotic and sent me home with painkillers. 'It will pass in a few days.'

It passed slowly, but it did pass.

The next weekend I was a lot better and went on a trip to celebrate my dad's sixtieth birthday. I was so looking forward to this. Andy would look after the children while I got to go to Belgium on my own! I was so excited.

I was delighted to see Carine there as well. It was only the second time since we had met in England but we talked as if we had known each other forever. It was a lovely day full of laughter and chats.

At one particular moment we were sitting outside in the sun, I felt a light chilly breeze. It felt good to be in the fresh air. I mentioned to Carine that I had felt when about five weeks pregnant that the baby's soul had come down to its body. She said she found that very early, but we didn't pay any attention to this. She said she was sure it was a girl, she felt the strong female energy.

Later that day, as we were having a last drink, we were standing with a small group when I suddenly felt an enormous tiredness in my tummy. It seemed very heavy and I felt worried. I could feel worry in my tummy. As I felt this, Carine obviously felt something was going on and asked me straight away if I needed to sit down. A funny little moment, that was.

One of our other conversations was a bit different. She said how she could feel something was about to happen. I would be needed as a healer. Everyone in my family in Belgium would be in a right panic, but I would have to be strong, push everything away, trust and heal. I could not place this vision at all and know now it was my own daughter's extremely premature birth.

The day after the party, I had an appointment to have a blood test. Even though the pain in my throat had gone as I was in Belgium I thought I would have everything checked. It was a Sunday, but thanks to knowing the doctor, this was possible. It was just to check all the general things and CMV, toxoplasmosis...

My father sent me the results when I was back in the UK. Those papers with weird words and numbers are like Chinese to me, I am not a medical person so didn't have a clue what they meant. I asked my dad but he too didn't have a clue. All he said was that he was sure that if there was a problem, the doctor would have contacted me personally. There were several red numbers on the results and, as anyone knows, red numbers are not a good sign. I sat there thinking about this but eventually let it go, trusting that the doctor would have called me if a problem had been detected... I would find out later that problems in the pregnancy were fully detected on the blood test but the doctor simply hadn't taken any notice.

On Wednesday 16th of May, 23 weeks + 1 day pregnant, I became aware of thick discharge when going to the toilet. The heaviness felt quite unusual. I mentioned this to Andy, but of course, he didn't have a clue what it could mean. I didn't want to be one of those over worried mums so I just kept an eye on it without telling anyone. The following three days, the discharge kept coming. My pelvis felt heavier and I noticed I had started to 'wobble' as one does at the end of a pregnancy when the baby descends into the pelvis. When I mentioned this to other people they just said it was normal as it was my fourth child. It felt different, though. I didn't really trust what was going on. My breasts felt less tense as if they were 'shrinking' again. That was very unusual, it had never happened before. Normally my breasts stayed firm and full until birth and a lot longer if breastfeeding followed.

It was then Saturday, so I planned to go and see the midwife after the weekend. I turned to the Belline cards once again and asked what was the state of the baby. The answer was once again: '17 Disease'. By now I was freaking out, but still kind of ignoring it, hoping the cards were wrong.

Saturday 19th of May, 23 weeks + 4 days pregnant. There was a big football match on TV. Champions league Bayern Munchen–Chelsea. Now this doesn't mean anything to me, but Andy loves football and is a big life-long Chelsea fan. He had a friend, Ewerton, coming over to watch the game with him. The children had gone to bed and we were preparing some dips and drinks in the kitchen when my pelvis felt very heavy and uncomfortable. I was standing there, watching them being silly and making jokes, rocking my hips from left

The Healing of the 1lb Baby

to right. I said to Andy: 'Goodness, my body feels tired, it's like I'm at the end of the pregnancy'. I knew this was not how I was meant to feel at this time in the pregnancy.

Andy suggested I should go to bed and rest and see the doctor on Monday if I was so worried.

Having had three full-term pregnancies, it seemed logical that I should not expect problems this time. This was Andy's view and who could blame him. He had not experienced the card readings and the visions I had!

After the throat pain, I had very short flashes of having a very premature baby. I kept telling myself to 'shut up'. My sister had had a baby born at only 25 weeks' gestation years earlier and I remembered very well what a struggle that had been, and I wasn't even 25 weeks yet. This could not happen, despite my pre-feelings.

Sunday 20th of May, 23 weeks + 5 days pregnant. As usual, we were up early – six o'clock – the joy of having three spirited young children! I felt cramps in my lower belly as if I were going to have my period. I went back upstairs to put on some clothes. I remember noticing again how 'normal' my breasts had become and not hard as they are when pregnant. Upstairs we had carpets in the bedrooms. I walked to Andy's side of the bed to get something when I suddenly had uncontrollable weeing. I tried to stop it and thought my pelvic floor wasn't very good that I couldn't keep my wee up any more! But that wasn't the case. Water was slowly but surely coming out of me, leaking onto the carpet. When the realization came that I was probably losing the amniotic, I panicked. I held my tummy as if to hold the baby in so she wouldn't 'fall out'. I kept praying in a quiet, whimpering voice: 'Please, please, Angels, help us, please help, she is too small, don't make me lose my baby, please, please help'. All the previous visions kind of slapped me in the face at the same time. We had come to that moment when somewhere I knew what was going to happen. I walked to the toilet very carefully, holding my belly. The water was still slowly running out in big drips, leaving a trail on the carpet. I sat on the toilet for a few minutes trying to think, while sobbing and praying, trying to comprehend what was going on.

My hands were trembling and my whole body was shivering.

I put on some clothes and walked downstairs, trying to support my body weight on my arms, to avoid downward shocks from the walking.

I told Andy I thought I had lost the amniotic. It had stopped running but I knew what had happened upstairs. I wanted to go for a check-up, right now. Andy didn't fully comprehend the seriousness of the situation as he was insisting on preparing breakfast for the children before we could go. I felt the occasional 'blub' of something coming out of me. I had no contraction and felt the baby move, which was comforting for both of us in a way. I noticed how undisturbed Andy appeared; he kept organizing things until I firmly told him that I really wanted to go NOW! Ewerton got worried as well and insisted that Andy should take me to the hospital immediately and he would look after the boys. We took Orla-Jane as she was only 21 months old and we thought she would be happier coming with us.

I hardly moved in the car, as I was scared that any movement would lead to contractions or the baby coming out.

Once we arrived at the hospital, Andy dropped me off so I could go in while he was looking for a parking space.

Chapter 4: Three scary days in the unknown

I walked hunched forward, still holding my stomach, worried that every step could trigger the baby's arrival. As I walked into the hospital, I had no idea where to go. It was the right department but there were doors and hallways in all directions. I sat down on the first chair I could find and luckily a mother and her pregnant daughter walked down the hallway and I asked them where the delivery department was. It was urgent, because my waters had broken and I was only 23 weeks pregnant. I could see the shock and fear on their faces and they helped me along. I pressed the bell and someone let me in. Right in front of me was the reception desk. I went straight towards it saying that my waters had broken and I was only 23 weeks pregnant and that I was very worried and would like to see someone. My voice was weak and trembled. The receptionist asked me if I had telephoned before I came. I said no, and she replied that I should have called before coming in. There I was in panic with a baby in my tummy that probably wouldn't be able to live if she came now and she dared to tell me that I should have called!!!!! If I had had the strength my actions might have been not very friendly. However, I managed to keep my mouth shut. I needed a doctor and quick!!

Luckily I was taken through quite quickly to an examination room. By the time I was in the room, Andy had arrived with Orla-Jane. It felt so good to just lie down and relax. First the nurse came in to take a blood sample, then the doctor followed. He was an older, Indian man, calm, reserved but friendly. Andy was standing at the window with Orla-Jane and the doctor advised he should draw her attention to what was outside as she might become distressed if she saw a stranger doing something to Mummy. I had never thought about it that way, but what he was saying made perfect sense. The doctor didn't say a lot, all he said was that it was indeed amniotic fluid I was losing and that we now had to be very careful that the baby wasn't infected. The fact that I didn't have any contractions was very good. I felt as if there was hope.

I was transferred to a room with two other ladies. We had to wait for the results of the test but I was given antibiotics straight away. Andy went home with Orla-Jane to pack a bag as we didn't have a clue what would happen next or how long I would be there.

The patient lying opposite me had apparently gone through a great deal to become pregnant and was now risking having a premature birth, so had been in hospital for several weeks. She unloaded her whole story. The energy these drama stories carry is enormous and so heavy. No wonder people need to tell someone. Afterwards the story teller feels good, but the listener ends up carrying the storyteller's burden. So, indeed, while I was lying there I sent her healing energy. I gave her burden of miscarriages, extremely premature births and stillborn babies back, with love and healing. None of us has to carry someone else's problems. No, this is not selfish. When someone is pouring out their problems, protect yourself. Imagine you are standing in a balloon of light. On the outside of the balloon there is a band of sparkling white light, green light and purple light. With an imaginary hand movement, and using a goodwill thought message, move the problem package back to them with green light, which is the healing colour. In this way, you are there as a listening ear, but do not take over the burden package from someone else.

The nurse on the ward that day was very short and had no communication skills whatsoever! Now, I am a foreigner in England and people should live wherever they like or feel at home, but if you have a job where communication is needed, you should speak the language. As I said, I am foreigner in the UK but I speak English, but I didn't have any idea what she was saying. She had a very heavy accent, rambled on and every time she said something I had to ask her to repeat it, her English was so poor. After a while she became bad tempered because I kept asking her to repeat what she had said. I eventually apologized and blamed myself, saying that I was from Belgium and didn't always understand everything... I didn't feel looked after at all. I was worried sick lying in that bed. In the meantime I had already called my mum in Belgium to let her know what was going on. We had a friend in Belgium who had lost her waters when pregnant and ended up having to lie flat in the hospital for months but at the end there was a healthy baby. So everyone on the other side of the Channel gave good advice: stay in bed and lie still! As we were unsure what would happen next, it was comforting to realize my family were thinking of me. They even suggested I should be transported to Belgium, because they were confident that I would receive good care there. They meant well, of course, but seemed to forget I was living in a well developed country and the hospital staff knew what they were doing.

I asked that nurse if I could walk to the toilet because every time I stood up, I felt water oozing out and heaviness in my lower abdomen. Also at this time I began having light cramps.

I was given pain killers and told I could walk to the toilet but if there was a problem, the alarm bell should be rung immediately. I was very uncomfortable returning to bed, but it was like heaven once there.

I was given special socks to prevent blood clots.

It was Sunday night, Andy came back with a bag of clothes and reading material. I was just in the middle of a course in Crystal therapy, so it would be the perfect learning material to keep me occupied. The nurse returned and said she was going to give me steroids to ripen the lungs of the baby, just in case of an early birth. This would enable the lungs to work better if birth was extremely premature. Apart from seeing the doctor who had confirmed I was losing my waters and receiving a blood test, I was left alone for some time, which made me very anxious.

The 'butcher-nurse' stuck this massive needle in my bum cheek. It hurt like hell, I was crying, begging her to stop. She told me in no uncertain terms to just deal with it, it was good for the baby and I would be fine. Any sign of empathy or reassurance was just non-existent.

I just sat there, in the unknown. Turning was uncomfortable, I could feel the baby's movements a lot harder, the movement of the baby felt a lot more rough against the inside of my tummy. I spoke to the baby, please be OK, and I thought, bloody hell will I have to lie here for four months? I needed a break, I've been given a break.

Monday 21st of May 2012. So here I was in a medium size hospital not having a clue what was going on, but glad I was still pregnant! Another day forward. A scan was scheduled. I was collected by the same nurse, who said we should go downstairs for the scan. She proceeded to get me to my feet. 'Do you expect me to walk?' I said. 'Yes, you'll be all right, don't worry,' she said.

The Healing of the 1lb Baby

She took me down the stairs, not even the elevator!!!!! I gingerly climbed down the stairs absolutely terrified, trying to hold back the tears, praying the baby would remain safely in the womb. With every step I just wanted to sit down, I wanted to cry and scream how scared I was, this just wasn't right. As we reached the lower floor I was greeted by a friendly young nurse. She looked at me in disbelief, obviously aware of my discomfort. 'Why is this lady walking down the stairs?' she asked. 'It looks as if it was too much for her.' She asked if I would like a wheelchair and brought one along. Thank you, Angel nurse!

As I was waiting for the scan, Andy came back. The boys were in school and, luckily, Orla-Jane had a place in nursery and they had already let us know that she could go every day for as long as necessary.

We didn't have to wait long. The ultrasonographer was very understanding and caring and helped me out of the wheelchair onto the table. Every movement felt too much and I felt a heavy aching in my abdomen.

And then we saw our little girl with hardly any supporting water left. Apart from the fact that the baby was alive and looked well on the scan, the ultrasonographer was not allowed to say anything. Andy went back to work and would return later.

Once I was back upstairs, the butcher nurse came in again with a massive, thick needle and the steroids. Pure agony! But I had to 'stop whining, it's for the baby'. Yes, fair enough, and in the whole turmoil of things I still didn't fully understand what was going on.

The same day I was taken to another examination room, away from butcher nurse. I still had light cramps but no one seemed to be paying any attention to this. It was slightly upsetting to be on a ward with heavily pregnant women, first one giving birth, others screaming as their babies came out, hearing babies' cries while I didn't know if my baby was going to live or…

Still, I had to walk to the toilet on my own; nobody seemed to care what was going on.

A different doctor came in to examine me. He asked me if I or my husband had had a different partner in the last few months... He didn't explain why he asked me this question. Even though I knew I hadn't been with anyone else since I met my husband and I trust my husband, still at that moment I started to doubt, which I really didn't need! Apparently it could have been linked to the infection. After this no one ever mentioned it again, luckily.

The doctor said he was really worried about the infection, the mucus plug and waters had gone, the baby was in danger.

I now had frequent light contractions but very irregularly. The nurse gave me more painkillers. I was praying for them to go away. There were moments when they became quite strong and they weren't just cramps but contractions. Everyone now kept a close eye on me; some lovely nurses, finally!

The neonatologist came in with a worried look on her face. With an Eastern European accent, she was a petite, blonde doctor with a friendly face. She stood at the bottom of my bed. She had come to explain what could happen. She explained that seeing as I had an infection and the waters had gone, there was nothing they could do. I was 23 weeks + 6 days pregnant. We could only pray for extra time to increase the baby's chance of survival. She explained (as I knew) that the baby was possibly too small or ill to survive. The steroids would give her a better chance. So far only half the dose had been administered. The seriousness of the situation was evident. At that time several big contractions occurred and I remember telling the neonatologist that if my baby wasn't well, I would not want them to save her. I felt that if she did arrive and was so ill, it would mean she didn't want to be here. I did not want a difficult life for her or my other children. Both the doctor and I had tears in our eyes.

The hospital only had facilities for babies born from 27 weeks onwards. If she came now, they would do their best.

But they would prefer to transfer her to the nearest hospital that handles extremely premature births.

I spoke to this little girl in my tummy and told her to, just for once, listen to me; she didn't ever have to listen to me again after this: 'Please stay in my tummy!'

As I asked her, I could feel that 'my demand' wasn't a good idea, something not good was going on.

The examination showed that there was no opening yet, which was great news. I was given a private room. How nice was this! So many thoughts were running through my mind. I called Andy to let him know the latest news. He promised to return that day after work when the children were in bed.

Several times that day, a nurse came in to check my blood pressure and see how I felt. The contractions had eased and the nurse brought me a bed pan so I didn't have to get up. Good, this was OK, I began to feel more settled and relaxed.

My third dose of steroids was given by a different nurse. I told her how horribly painful they were. She said it depended how they were given. If the steroid dose is pressed in slowly, the pain is minimized. And so it happened – no pain, thanks to this sensible nurse.

Chapter 5: Transfer

Around 21.30 a nurse and a doctor came in to tell me that an ambulance would transfer me to a hospital where better equipment was available for very premature babies. It was the best decision that doctor ever made as we will discover later. I am forever grateful!

Only 30 minutes later two very friendly paramedics appeared with a stretcher.

One was in his forties, the other about thirty. He was very cheeky and his presence cleared the tense atmosphere. Then a very lively young midwife appeared and in a cheery voice said she would accompany me in the ambulance to the next hospital.

At this stage no one seemed to know where the other hospital was located. Someone mentioned that it was a four hour journey away. I panicked, realizing I did not have enough clothing with me and Andy would not be able to visit. I was assured all would be dealt with once we were there.

Before the ambulance left, I called Andy about the transfer and told him I would telephone him once I arrived.

The Healing of the 1lb Baby

The ambulance men were making jokes and everyone was laughing, which was nice. I managed a smile. It made me forget why I was being transferred. They helped me on to the stretcher. I asked them how they did this with bigger people. The stretcher was very narrow, and as I am a petite lady and wasn't very comfortable, how do they do it? The younger guy joked that they 'just flap the loose overhanging bits up and fold it together on top of the stretcher'. This made me laugh, as my imagination ran riot. I know this is not particularly funny, but it was good to lighten up a little.

And off we went, two guys, a lady and me, all together in the ambulance. The midwife was sitting next to me reading. I just closed my eyes for a while. It had been another hectic day. The contractions and cramps had stopped, although I felt some pressure on my bladder every time I moved. It wasn't exactly the most comfortable trip. The ambulance men put the address in the GPS and saw that it would be a good two hour journey. One asked the other if they should put on the siren. They decided to wait until it was busy or necessary. It felt like we were driving in a straight line, as there was no traffic, thanks to the time of the day. The reason I had to travel so far was because local hospitals who dealt with extremely premature babies had no beds available. But again, it was meant to be, as I found out later.

I was only able to doze on and off. I had my hands on my tummy, feeling the baby; she was still moving, that was good.

We finally arrived in another part of the country. Everyone was happy we had arrived safe and sound with baby inside. I hadn't quite realized until we arrived that the midwife had been with me in case the baby had been born during the journey. The ambulance guys were having a little stretch while the midwife put all her stuff away, including a tiny, pink 5.5-cm diameter hat. She showed it to me and said in a positive manner, 'Well, luckily we didn't need this'. She meant well but for me it was shocking. I didn't have a clue how small my baby still was. I only knew she was too small, but I had never seen a baby of 23–24 weeks before. I just swallowed and gave a vague smile.

When they wheeled me out, everyone was very impressed with the hospital. It was big and light and looked new or had been renovated. It felt good. Hopefully, the people would be nice as well! When in hospital, you are so submissive and reliant upon the staff and it is important they are there for you.

We took the lift upstairs to the delivery department. They had been expecting me.

The midwife helped me onto the bed and all three of them said goodbye and wished me the best of luck.

A lovely nurse took over. She took my blood pressure and a blood sample; a doctor would examine me in the morning.

The room had four beds and mine was the first on the right next to the bathroom. I felt safe.

Tuesday 22nd of May

When I woke up the next morning I felt good. I settled down to study my course on Crystal therapy which I had brought with me. I had all that time to read! I paid for the TV and was fine. Andy wouldn't be able to come today as it wasn't an easy combination for him. He was running his business and looking after three children. Luckily, there was school and nursery in the daytime but school finished at three so that would cut Andy's day very short. My whole family lived in Belgium and we only had Andy's parents to help out. Even though both are in their eighties, they jumped in and this was a massive help. Andy sent me pictures via his phone of the kiddies. They were missing Mummy because I was always there. It was so confusing for them. Andy would visit the next day, Wednesday.

All the necessary steroids had been given and now every extra day was a plus.

I was told several times by the doctor how small the chances were of a baby surviving at this level of gestation and the potential problems that could arise. I was listening but not really taking it in; my baby would be fine, they had to stop being so negative. Was it ignorance or stupidity? I called it positivity, I don't know.

I was given a bed on the ward with full-term expectant mums. Watching them battle with contractions and then being wheeled off to the delivery room was quite difficult to deal with. One of the expectant mums was lying in the bed beside me. She and her husband were excited and they consumed chips before she was eventually taken away to be induced. My three previous births had been normal, but I can imagine if there were problems with the baby or pregnancy and it was the first time, how sad it would be hearing other people's happiness.

Suddenly the door opened and a distressed lady appeared who was 25 weeks pregnant. She was followed by a concerned number of people who I assumed were her family. Soon the room was filled with noisy relatives all talking at once, while the woman screamed for her baby. She was having contractions. I found this most distressing and my fears for the safety of my own baby multiplied by the second. I kept telling myself, 'this is not happening to me, it is not happening to me, it is someone else, please help this lady'. To add to the chaos another young girl arrived experiencing contractions, who apparently knew the whole family. The noise gathered momentum as she shouted above everyone that her boyfriend had been in a fight, arrested and then admitted to hospital. It was like a circus!

Eventually both ladies left, I don't know where they went, and peace was restored.

While all this was happening, I had a few concerning contractions but the painkillers helped. I hadn't been examined since the previous Sunday. I was wondering when they would check me again.

I found it difficult to turn around as my belly felt very heavy, I hardly dared move or go to the toilet; my tummy had shrunk and looked small and my breast size was back to normal. I felt the baby move so that was a comfort.

On that day, Andy and I decided to let the family know that we were expecting a baby girl and that her name would be Elouisa. We felt it would be right for the family to know who to pray for.

Four years earlier my sister had had a baby born at 25 weeks. This would be her second time 'digesting' that experience, and it would possibly bring back many painful memories.

Chapter 6: Energetically explained reasons for premature birth and pregnancy problems

- Infection
- Preeclampsia
- Growth restriction
- Placental abruption
- Cervical problems
- Preterm premature rupture of membranes
- Fertility treatments and link to higher chance of pregnancy and delivery problems
- Spontaneous premature birth

1. Chakras

For whatever reason, premature birth or pregnancy problems are caused by blockages in the energy system. Further information about the chakras gives insight in these blockages. Very often it will be noticed that several physical problems have occurred in the past as a sign of the blockage before the premature birth or pregnancy problems happened. One thing repeats itself every time and that is, whatever problem occurs during pregnancy, the Sacral chakra shows a blockage.

Pregnancy problems and premature birth = blocked Sacral chakra/energy point of creativity, emotions and sexuality. Depending on the exact pregnancy problem, it is explained which other chakra/energy point(s) are blocked and can than be referred to in the list of chakras below.

1.1 Base chakra/connection with Mother Earth/first chakra
- Situated between our anus and genitals; it is connected to our coccyx and opens downwards
- The chakra of grounding/connection to Mother Earth
- Sense: Smell
- Colour: Red

A healthy Base chakra creates:
- Survival
- Security
- Physical will of existence
- Confidence
- Trust
- Enjoyment of the incarnation and earthly life
- The right to be

A blocked Base chakra creates:
- Fear
- Uncertainty
- Little or no psychological and physical resistance

Addictions linked to the Base chakra:
- Gambling
- Shopping
- Working
- Food

- Compulsive behaviour

Our Base chakra can get blocked by the following:
- Birth trauma
- Physical and emotional abuse
- Inherited traumas of parents
- Serious surgery or severe illness
- Long treatment, doctor/hospital
- Poor physical bond with mother
- Rape
- Physical violence or violent environment
- Abandonment and physical neglect
- Malnutrition or problems with feeding
- First time on Earth/reincarnated Angels

Physical disorders that can occur caused by a blockage of this chakra:
- Chilblains
- Parkinson's disease
- Osteoporosis
- Anaemia
- Panic attacks
- Anxiety
- Appendix
- Nail biting
- Kidney stones
- Constipation/diarrhoea
- Bladder problems
- No stress resistance
- Insomnia
- Athlete's foot
- Disorders of feet, legs, guts, bones, knees
- Financial worries and problems
- Low blood pressure
- Allergies
- Eating disorders
- Lower back pain

- Obesity
- Compulsive behaviour/ticks
- Cerebral palsy
- Haemorrhoids
- Hyperactivity

1.2 Sacral chakra/ second chakra
- Situated in the bottom part of our Holy bone; it opens upwards above the genitals
- Sense: Taste
- Colour: Orange

A healthy Sacral chakra creates:
- Sexuality
- Propagation
- Creativity
- Self consciousness
- Emotions
- The right to feel

A blocked Sacral chakra creates:
- Guilt

Addictions linked to the Sacral chakra:
- Sex
- Alcohol
- Heroin

Our Sacral chakra can get blocked by the following events:
- Inherited traumas of parents around sexuality
- Rejection
- Alcoholic families
- Religious or moral severity against lust
- Sexual and physical abuse
- Emotional violence
- Emotional manipulation
- Any situation linked to emotional stress

- Personality severaly stifled by parents
- Unstable situation
- Neglect

Physical problems that can occur caused by a blockage of this chakra:
- Mood swings
- Periods staying away/menstruation problems
- Thrush
- Prostate problems
- Problems with the male sexual organ
- Nosebleeds
- Leukaemia
- Cancer of uterus and ovaries
- Early menopause
- Fertility problems
- Middle back pain
- Disorders or problems with: Semen, urine, blood, lymph
- Premature delivery
- Infections
- Obesity
- Preeclampsia
- Disorders of the uterus and ovaries
- High cholesterol
- Glandular problems
- PMS

1.3 Solar Plexus/ third chakra
- Situated 2 cm above the belly button; it opens forwards
- Sense: Seeing
- Colour: Yellow

A healthy Solar Plexus creates:
- Will
- Good self esteem

- Strength
- Self control
- The right to act

A blocked Solar Plexus creates:
- Shame
- Prejudice

Addictions linked to the Solar Plexus:
- Cocaine
- Caffeine
- Work
- Rage
- Amphetamines

Our Solar Plexus can get blocked by the following:
- Shame
- Guilt
- Authoritarian practices
- Uncertain situations
- Suppression of the will
- Physical abuse
- Hazardous surroundings
- Fear of punishment
- Emotional manipulation
- Responsibilities that are not age-appropriate
- Parents' inherited shame

Physical disorders that can occur caused by a blockage of this chakra:
- Malfunctions of the stomach, liver, pancreas, gallbladder, kidneys
- Psoriasis
- Chronic fatigue
- Selfishness
- Lupus
- Fever

- Acid reflux
- Stomach inflammation
- Digestive disorders
- Eating disorders
- Ulcers
- Diabetes
- Pimples
- Conjunctivitis
- Cellulite
- Muscle cramps
- Muscle disorders
- Parkinson's disease
- Warts
- High blood pressure
- Motion sickness
- Anger
- Obesity
- Preeclampsia
- High cholesterol
- Bronchitis
- Cold sores
- Hyperactivity

1.4. Heart chakra/fourth chakra
- Situated at the heart level in the middle of our chest; it opens forwards
- Sense: Seeing
- Colour: Green

A healthy Heart chakra creates:
- Relationships
- Balance
- Love
- Intimacy
- The right to love and be loved

A blocked Heart chakra creates:

- Grief
- Sadness

Addictions linked to the Heart chakra:
- Tobacco
- Sugar
- Love
- Marijuana

Our Heart chakra can get blocked by the following:
- Non-recognized grief
- Loss
- Embarrassment
- Rejection, abandonment
- Acquired grief of parents
- Separation
- Death of a loved one
- Loveless and cold environment
- Conditional love
- Sexual or physical violence
- Betrayal

Physical disorders that can occur caused by blockage of this chakra:
- Allergies and hypersensitivity
- Stutter
- Psoriasis
- Sunken chest
- Disorders of the heart, lungs, thymus, breasts and arms
- Problems with blood circulation
- Asthma
- A weak immune system
- Lung/breathing problems
- Shooting/sharp pains between shoulder blades
- Pain in the chest
- Anorexia and bulimia

- Skin disorders
- A desire for plastic surgery
- Heavy coughs/bronchitis

1.5 Throat chakra/fifth chakra
- Situated in the throat, it opens forwards
- Sense: Hearing
- Colour: Blue

A healthy Throat chakra creates:
- Communication
- Mental energy
- Inspiration
- Independence
- Truth
- The right to hear the truth and to speak the truth

A blocked Throat chakra creates:
- Lies

Addictions linked to the Throat chakra:
- Opiates
- Marijuana

Our Throat chakra can get blocked by the following:
- Authoritarian parents
- Lies
- Verbal abuse
- Excessive criticism

Physical problems that can occur caused by a blockage of this chakra:
- Diseases of the mouth and teeth
- Nosebleeds
- Stutter
- Rigid jaws

- Throat complaints, deafness, stiff neck
- Weak neck
- Sensitivity to ringing in the ears
- Common colds and throat infections
- Hoarseness, voice loss, sore throat
- Shoulder area is tense
- Lump in the throat
- Disorders of throat, ears, voice and neck
- Thyroid problems
- Asthma
- Sinusitis
- Mumps
- Gum disease
- Cold sores

2. Infection

A human with an infection has another organism inside them, which gets its nourishment from that person. It colonizes that person and reproduces inside them. The human with that organism (germ) inside is called the host.

It is only an infection if the colonization harms the host. It uses the host to feed on and multiplies at the expense of the host to such an extent that his/her health is affected.

Any kind of systemic inflammation or infection can cause a mother to have her baby early, including infections in the mouth, such as gum disease – refer to 1.2 and 1.5; vagina or uterus – refer to 1.2; and kidneys – refer to 1.2 and 1.3.

Toxoplasmosis, CMV and Streptococcus B all have their seat in a blocked Sacral chakra. Refer to 1.2.

Streptococcus A: A throat infection is seated in a blocked Sacral and Throat chakra. Refer to 1.2 and 1.5.

3. Preeclampsia

Preeclampsia is a condition that can appear very unexpectedly during pregnancy and can cause a dramatic turn in a pregnancy. It is the highest cause of death in pregnant women. Some women need to have their babies delivered prematurely to avoid this condition becoming life-threatening. This illness is of course a threat to the unborn child too.

During pregnancy the volume of blood increases by almost half, while the blood pressure somewhat decreases. In the case of preeclampsia the blood volume remains normal (i.e. non-pregnancy level '... the blood volume does not increase), and the blood vessels pull together, causing the blood pressure to rise. The cause of this abnormal phenomenon is medically not fully known, but it is likely to do with an abnormal construction of the blood vessels at the point where the placenta is attached to the uterus. In addition, the endothelium, the cell layer that coats the inside of the blood vessels, does not work properly. It is suspected that it secretes substances that go against the normal adjustment of the blood circulation during pregnancy. The lack of adjustment of the blood circulation leads to a reduced blood flow in the placenta, kidney, liver and brain. This will affect the functioning of these organs, causing all sorts of problems. In the worst case, the placenta may come loose, the kidneys fail, a convulsive seizure (similar to an epileptic seizure) could occur; there may be bleeding in the liver and brain, moisture may accumulate in the lungs, etc. These complications may eventually prove fatal. The lowered blood supply to the baby can cause lack of oxygen and lead to severe growth retardation.

Problems can occur at various times in pregnancy, and they tend to worsen and expand. In most cases, luckily, the problems remain limited. The later in the pregnancy preeclampsia pops up, the greater the chance of bringing a healthy child into the world. The more developed the child is, the fewer disadvantages it faces. Even a sudden and fiercely developing preeclampsia is less threatening for mother and child when there is rapid intervention. Other health problems, e.g. existing kidney problems or diabetes, will, of course, be complicated by the evolution and approach of preeclampsia.

The condition cannot be medically cured at present, but can be kept under control with the right treatment. If recognized early, there is a higher assurance of maximal guarantee for the health of the mother, and the baby can be born under the best conditions in the world.

There are no unique features from which one can infer preeclampsia. Potential signs are: headaches, vomiting and abdominal pain. If the symptoms are slight they may not be recognized as a sign of preeclampsia and they are sometimes attributed to other illnesses. This can be a problem. A very belated recognition often makes it impossible to do anything to treat the condition. Immediate delivery of the baby sometimes has to be carried out to save the lives of mother and baby.

Some symptoms can ring an alarm bell and can easily be recognized by pregnant women themselves. The occurrence of nausea and vomiting during the second half of a pregnancy is abnormal. In that case a doctor should be consulted and a thorough check for preeclampsia carried out. Problems with urination – darkening of the urine, sudden need to urinate or being able to urinate only a little – point to kidney problems. A severe pain in the upper right abdomen, nausea and vomiting may indicate serious liver problems. Some signs can only be detected if regular monitoring is done by a physician. In order to know whether the changes have any meaning, the doctor needs to know how the situation was at the beginning of the pregnancy, or even better, before the pregnancy. Elevated blood pressure (hypertension), especially after the twentieth week of pregnancy, is an important indicator of preeclampsia. However, one should not focus too exclusively on hypertension as a number of pregnant women who develop preeclampsia do not have high blood pressure.

Growth retardation is an indication of a serious problem and can be detected by ultrasound. Protein in the urine can also ring alarm bells. When signs of preeclampsia are already established in a woman – headache, nausea, visual disturbances, etc. – it indicates something is not right. When such symptoms are detected it is best that a doctor is contacted immediately.

The cause of preeclampsia is not fully understood. However, it is thought that the placenta does not develop properly because of a problem with the blood vessels supplying it. The placenta is the organ that links the mother's blood supply to her unborn baby's blood supply. Nutrients and oxygen pass through the placenta from mother to baby. Waste products can pass from the baby back into the mother. To support the growing baby, the placenta needs a large and constant supply of blood from the mother. In preeclampsia, the placenta does not get enough blood. This could be because the placenta did not develop properly when it was forming during the first half of the pregnancy.

This problem with the placenta means that the blood supply between mother and baby is disrupted. Signals from the damaged placenta affect the mother's blood vessels, causing high blood pressure. At the same time, problems in the kidneys may cause valuable proteins that should remain in the mother's blood to leak into her urine, resulting in protein in the urine (proteinuria).

Now, as given in this medical explanation, the following physical causes and problems related to this condition are:

- Blood problems (Sacral chakra)
- Protein in urine (Sacral chakra)
- Problems with urine/urination (Sacral chakra)
- Problems with kidneys (Solar Plexus)
- Problems with the liver (Solar Plexus)
- Diabetes (Solar Plexus)
- Nausea/vomiting (Solar Plexus)
- High blood pressure (Solar Plexus)
- Blood circulation (Heart chakra)

The reason why this phenomenon causes illness in pregnancy is that it is linked with problems of the blood and urine. These physical problems can occur when the Sacral chakra gets blocked. Women who get preeclampsia also suffer from a blocked Solar Plexus and Heart chakra. Refer to 1.2, 1.3 and 1.4.

When the blockages are severe and create illness, it normally means that certain events from past lives and family circles are carried heavily in the energy system and it has become too much. Past life healing and family circle breaking during chakra healing is always deeper than healing purely on current life-events and the results are more profound.

4. Growth restrictions/Premature birth

The following are different reasons, which depend on the mother's habits, for growth restrictions/premature birth of the baby.

Growth restrictions/premature birth can be caused by:

4.1 Alcohol during pregnancy: The mother has a blocked Sacral chakra. Refer to 1.2.

4.2 Infection: The mother has a blocked Sacral chakra and another blocked energy point, depending on the type of infection, as fully explained in point 2 above.

4.3 Smoking during pregnancy: This has an effect on the blood vessels that can make the baby lighter. The blood flow to the placenta is cut down. Very often babies born to mothers who smoked during pregnancy have less well developed lungs. The mother has blocked Sacral and Heart chakras. Refer to 1.2 and 1.4.

These physical disorders/blockages in the mother can be carried on to the unborn child. This is called a family circle blockage and will be explained later on.

4.4 Stress and high blood pressure: The high blood pressure leads to a reduced blood flow to the uterus and placenta;

this diminishes the baby's supply of nutrients, which causes it to be smaller and lighter. The mother has blocked Base and Sacral chakras and Solar Plexus. Refer to 1.1, 1.2 and 1.3.

4.5 Under-eating in the mother/nutritional problems: The mother has blocked Base and Heart chakras. Refer to 1.1 and 1.4.

4.6 Chromosome aberrations: The baby has a blocked Base chakra; karmic, unfinished business between child and parents; the baby decided to come this way.

4.7 Disproportionate (asymmetric) growth restriction: The body of the baby is too small and the proportions are not normal. The belly is proportionally smaller than the other body parts. This kind of slowdown is most commonly seen in reduced efficiency of the placenta. The mother has a blocked Sacral chakra; refer to 1.2. The baby has blocked Base and Sacral chakras; refer to 1.1 and 1.2.

4.8 Babies born via caesarean section: The child has a blocked Base chakra (1.1) and knows a lot of fear. If the mother demands a caesarean section without its being needed, she has a blocked Base chakra (1.1) and knows many fears.

5. Placental abruption

A placental abruption is a serious condition in which the placenta partially or completely separates from the uterus before the baby is born. The condition can deprive the baby of oxygen and nutrients, and cause severe bleeding that can be dangerous to both mother and child. A placental abruption also increases the risk of the baby having growth problems (if the abruption is small and goes unnoticed), be born prematurely or be stillborn. Placental abruption happens in about one in 150 pregnancies. It's most common in the third trimester but can happen any time after twenty weeks.

In most cases, some vaginal bleeding, ranging from a

small amount to an obvious and sudden gush, will occur. Sometimes, though, the blood stays in the uterus behind the placenta, so bleeding might not be noticed at all. Most women will have some uterine tenderness or lower back pain. And in close to a quarter of cases, an abruption will cause the woman to go into labour prematurely.

This condition is linked to blocked Base and Sacral chakras. Refer to 1.1 and 1.2.

6. Cervical problems

Insufficient cervix, such as one that is weak, thin and short, increases the risk of preterm birth.

Incompetent cervix is a condition in which a woman's cervix begins to open, or dilate, in the second trimester of pregnancy. The cervix is called 'incompetent' because it isn't able to stay closed long enough to allow a pregnancy to reach full term.

If an incompetent cervix is diagnosed in a pregnant woman, many physicians will place a cerclage or a stitch in the cervix, to help it stay closed until the baby is fully developed. Women who suffer from this condition have energetically blocked Base and Sacral chakras, Solar Plexus and Heart chakra. Refer to 1.1, 1.2, 1.3 and 1.4.

7. Preterm premature rupture of membranes

This is a condition where the membranes, for no reason, rupture. As a result the baby is open to infection and has no amniotic fluid. Very often it will cause labour to start. As with cervical problems, it is caused by a blockage in the Base and Sacral chakras, Solar Plexus and Heart chakra. Refer to 1.1, 1.2, 1.3 and 1.4.

8. Fertility treatments

When fertility treatments are needed, it means there was already an obvious blockage in the Sacral chakra in either the man or the woman. If the fertility problem is with the man, once the woman becomes pregnant via fertility treatment, the pregnancy will proceed smoothly, provided the woman has no energy blockage.

What might happen is that, because she has put so much pressure on herself because this baby is so important and because it has been difficult to conceive, the woman creates fear and uncertainty in herself and the baby (this happens unconsciously) so she will end up needing a caesarean.

If the reason for fertility treatment lies with the woman, there is a very high chance that the pregnancy or labour will cause problems as well. The reason for this is a blocked Sacral chakra. This blockage will not go away once pregnancy begins and fertility treatment may very often 'create' a multiple pregnancy, which is heavy on the human body if it hasn't happened naturally.

9. Spontaneous premature birth

There is no such thing as spontaneous premature birth; there is always an energetic reason for it to happen.

Apparently there is a genetic influence in having a (spontaneous) premature birth. This then is linked to the typical family circles.

We all owe our existence to energy, and we unconsciously take over energy blockages from the people who care for us – parents, grandparents, carers… Why? Because we are all connected. We choose where we will be born and whom we will meet in order to learn the lessons our soul needs to learn. If your mother and grandmothers have a history of a certain type of premature delivery, there is a high chance that you will have taken over that particular blocked energy centre (this is called a family circle) and therefore also a high chance that you will have the same pregnancy or delivery problems.

Breaking family circles, without feeling guilty towards the family, because guilt shows a blockage in the Sacral chakra (seat of the emotions), is so liberating! It offers you the chance to let go of past happenings, emotions, habits that keep coming back time and time again! It is necessary to cut the cords of family circles and live your life as whom you are. This way you also liberate your children from all of the baggage, so they can be whom they are without that massive rucksack!

This can be done with the help of a spiritual healer, past life regression, cord cutting or simply clearing your own energy system. You can learn more about this in my book *Heal by Intention – Crystal Learning and Oracle Cards*. The breaking of family circles can be a long process, step by step, but when it happens, beautiful and releasing.

9.1 Where and why does preterm birth happen?

Over sixty per cent of preterm births occur in Africa and South Asia, but preterm birth is truly a global problem. In the lower-income countries, on average, twelve per cent of babies are born too soon, compared with nine per cent in higher-income countries. Within countries, poorer families are at higher risk. The reason why is clear. Families with lower incomes very often have to deal with insecure, unstable situations, which have their seat in a blocked Sacral chakra (1.2). There is a lot more stress because of the insecurity (1.1) and very often shame for their situation (1.3).

Pregnancy problems and preterm birth happens more than ever. Why? Because many of us have lived many times before and been through many happenings which are still present in the energy system. We do 'forget' about all of this when we are born but it cannot be denied that it is still there! As many of these past and present lifetime events have/had to do with emotions or sexuality, this blockage occurs with more people than ever. Unfortunately, it is the energy point of reproduction which results in more and more fertility and pregnancy problems and preterm births. We have entered a time where it is all becoming too much. This causes the mind (even though the events are consciously forgotten) and the energy system to break down, and as a result illness is created, which is a cry for help! Luckily we have entered into an important time for living, where awareness is higher than ever and we can heal in the deepest levels of the subconscious, pull out the roots of the blockage, heal the mind and energy wheel and be restored to our natural state; this is possible for each of us – perfect health, whole love and full happiness.

*Part 2:
A new life begins;
Elouisa is born*

Chapter 7: Born at twenty-four weeks' pregnancy

It was Wednesday the 23rd of May and I was awake early. I felt quite chilled out and happy. Another day had arrived and my beautiful baby was still in my tummy. The contractions had faded completely. I had a lovely chat with Andy on the phone and he promised to come later with more clothes, treats and reading material. And yes, I was 24 weeks pregnant today! It was quiet on the ward and rather peaceful.

I had been constipated for four days and subconsciously felt unable to 'let go', for fear of triggering the onset of labour.

My stomach appeared to have shrunk, and as I stood up I was aware of a strong downward pressure.

I shuffled steadily to the bathroom and placed myself on the toilet. As I pushed I could feel release. Suddenly I felt as if I had defecated and there was complete release, only, nothing had happened. In a hundredth of a second I remembered the feeling when the head has finally fully descended during birth. I was shocked to discover when I looked in the mirror in front of me, a tiny head between my legs. I had just gently pushed my baby's head out. I trembled, my hands were shaking. My body was freezing cold. My fear stirred me into action. I gently held her little head with one hand and pulled the emergency cord with the other. Although I was trying to scream for help only a feeble cry escaped. A million thoughts rushed through my head, what if no one reacted to my emergency call! I walked to the door and opened it. I cried, 'Help, help, please, my baby is coming out'.

A young pregnant girl with long blonde hair took one look at me and jumped out of bed. She looked shocked and frightened and asked if she should get someone. 'Yes please, now, my baby is coming out.'

As she walked out of the room I left the door on the latch, and a midwife came in. She only needed to look at me once to see what was happening. She screamed that she needed the specialized team 'NOW, HEAD'S OUT!'

Two more midwives came flying in. They supported me and the third one, Laura, went on her knees in front of me. I was still standing, shaking like a leaf, crying uncontrollably and sobbing, 'It's too early, too early. She can't come out yet.' Laura comforted me and calmed me down. It was now up to me to push gently until the baby's body appeared. I didn't feel a thing.

After the birth Laura cut the cord. It was quiet. There was no crying. My eyes were shut tight. I was too afraid to look. She was taken straight away to the doctors of the NICU (Neonatal Intensive Care Unit), who were ready with all the necessary equipment. Whatever was going on, I knew that she was in the best possible place and would receive the best treatment.

I was so weak. I could hardly stand and through my tears I kept asking if she was alive. 'Yes,' said Laura, 'yes, she's alive and it is a girl, did you know?' 'Yes, a little girl, called Elouisa,' I replied. I was shaking, crying and felt completely powerless. I felt a deep sad emptiness, the tears were rolling over my cheeks and my nose was running too, a complete surrender. I felt no scruples or shame about myself, I had allowed my emotions full rein and all embarrassment went.

Now I didn't know what was going on with her. I still stood there, supported by two midwives and a third one on her knees 'between my legs'. She was waiting for the placenta to come. The midwives had decided to give me an injection to avoid bleeding but because the placenta was still so small it had cramped after receiving the injection and was refusing to come out. Laura gently tried to pull the cord but was afraid the cord might snap off and then the placenta would be stuck inside me. We stood there a while longer until the midwives decided to give it a rest and try again later.

They wiped my nose and tears, put me in a hospital gown and helped me into the bed they had prepared just outside the door. The place was heaving with people; eyes piercing into me all looking shocked and compassionate. I looked down and tried to ignore everyone around me. All I wanted was to crawl away deep under the sheets where no one could see me. Instead, I just laid on my back, my arms lifeless next to my body staring into nothing.

It was there and then, on that completely surrendered moment that something happened. I felt I was in a different time and space. As I was wheeled through the corridor to another room, an unexplained calm came over me and all my worry was over, everything was fine. Even though I had been sad only five minutes earlier, there was this inexplicable feeling of trust and knowing that Higher help was all around us.

The next procedure was the removal of the placenta. Two different midwives gently tried to pull the cord, but nothing happened. Their worst fears were realized when the cord snapped, leaving the placenta inside me. Now I would be handed over to the surgeon.

One of the midwives asked me if I wanted to call anyone. I asked her if she could call Andy. I felt embarrassment in a way, that I had put his baby in this position. I couldn't tell him she was born. When we had spoken an hour before all had been well; it was the news he least expected to hear.

When the midwife left the room I had two minutes to myself. The person I did call was Ann, the healer who had taught me so much over the years. I told her my baby Elouisa was born too early. She was quiet and I knew that was because she was 'looking, energetically, at Elouisa'. She said she couldn't see any problems. I said, 'But Ann, she weighs 535 grams!' 'Heal, Marie, trust and heal. She is fine.' My earlier feeling that all would be fine was confirmed. The capability to hold on to that trust was incredibly difficult, when I was being crashed to pieces by my ego whispering in my ear and all the medical facts from the doctors linked to a baby born that early.

The midwife came in again. Andy was on his way.

In a short while, I was wheeled to the operating theatre to have the placenta removed.

I hadn't seen or heard anything about Elouisa. I now had to be dealt with.

Luckily I did not have to be put to sleep completely. With an epidural in my back only my lower body was asleep. The anaesthetist was a young, good looking, funny, friendly man; he kept making jokes and made me feel very much at ease. By keeping the atmosphere light he made a world of difference. Job well done, mister anaesthetist! I didn't feel a thing and it all worked out very well and was over quickly. Before I even knew it my whole lower body was asleep. The doctor who directed the operation was female and friendly. I felt in safe hands, she made me feel comfortable and I knew I was going to be handled gently and with care. She then, with her hands and small tools removed the placenta. That happened vaginally so no knives were used or scarring caused and the procedure was natural. It felt as if my womb was emptied. Nothing was allowed to remain. Every piece was removed and put in a bucket to be brought to the lab for inspection. She said that the placenta was in quite a state, it fell completely apart, and that the infection had attacked the placenta and my baby. Via the cord, doctors can also check the stress level of the baby. Hers was lower than most full term babies. This had been to her advantage. She just simply came out, no stress, no worry. She had to, to save me and herself.

After the operation I was put in a fresh bed and wheeled to the recovery space, which appeared to be a separate area in a hallway blocked off with a curtain. Once the epidural had worn off, I would be able to go and see Elouisa.

I couldn't wait to feel my legs again. It felt very uncomfortable.

Andy arrived. No matter how 'good' and brave and 'OK' I had felt, the second I saw him, I broke down in tears. I felt like a little girl desperate for a long, warm cuddle and a shoulder to cry on.

Five minutes after Andy, the doctor came in with more information about Elouisa. He brought a picture of her as well, in a nice frame. Thinking about it now, this was probably just in case she didn't survive. I expect all parents are given a picture of their child to remember them by.

Elouisa looked very bruised and blue all over her body, especially her head, face and shoulders. 'She weighs 535 grams; just over one pound,' I was told.

She had tubes sticking out all over her. Here in this picture was our little girl.

I cried the second I held that picture. Sadness, guilt, fear, overwhelmed me and my breath faltered.

The doctor explained that it would take a few days before she could be called 'stable'. At this point, every hour was an hour forward. After two days it would be, every day is a day forward. Step by step. The doctor did not give us any really positive words.

The Healing of the 1lb Baby

He explained that we would have to wait and see what the bruising would do. These bruises are, effectively, bleeding on the inside of her body. She also had two small bleeds in the brain. We would have to wait and see how that would evolve.

As the doctor, who was very highly trained and experienced, was explaining, even though I realized he knew what he was talking about, I refused to allow this information to sink in or penetrate my mind. 'All of this will dissolve, she is fine!' I had to think this way. Over the following weeks/months, it would happen that I would suddenly think dark. What if I was being over positive, and un-realistic? Luckily I always found the strength to blow these thoughts out of my mind as quickly as they had entered.

My waters had been broken for 72 hours before Elouisa came out spontaneously. Whatever was left of amniotic fluid was clear.

When she was born, she was not breathing nor making any effort to breath, was smelly, pale and puss covered, but she was given inflation breaths. She improved and had a reasonable chest wall movement. She gasped and picked up. At that point she was moved to a transwarmer. Intubation was attempted, poor view during intubation caused by mucus in the trachea and suction was applied, followed by bagging. At seven minutes thirty seconds the intubation was successful. There was a good equal chest wall movement and air entry.

She was moved to the NICU department.

Andy went to see her on his own.

I had been given a single room, which was very much appreciated. He came back, half smiling half crying. A mixed emotion. To see his little girl alive, fighting like a bull, but so fragile looking at the same time.

'She is so small, so incredibly small, she fits in my hand,' he cried.

We hugged, a long, strong, deeply emotional hug.

The feeling in my legs started to return. I went in a wheelchair, still with a catheter attached to me. Andy, a nurse and a doctor brought me to see Elouisa for the first time. Andy prepared me again for how small she really was.

Are you ever prepared? No.

I was wheeled through the big automatic double doors of the NICU. The bleeps and lights were overwhelming. Everywhere were wires, computers and incubators. I had never been here before.

We all had to wash our hands thoroughly. This procedure was mandatory every time we entered the room from then on. Over the next few weeks my hands became red raw from washing.

'She's at the window – the best place,' Andy said.

My eyes were focused on the incubator at the window in the corner. I could feel other parents in the room looking at me, maybe remembering how they had felt seeing their baby for the first time. The nurse lowered the incubator. I was shocked by what I saw. I tried to hold back the tears as short sharp intakes of breath caught at me. I saw our baby. A microscopically small baby. I was not prepared.

'You can touch her,' said the nurse.

'No, I couldn't do that.' I was terrified.

'No, really, darling, it's okay, I touched her too,' said Andy. 'Just don't stroke her, her skin is too frail.'

Her skin was not fully formed yet, it was still sticky; a week later that would change.

I put my hands through the circles in the incubator and laid them upon her.

My anxiousness fell away. I said, 'Hello Elouisa, it's Mummy.' Andy placed his hand on my shoulder. Elouisa moved her leg.

I was assured I could come and see her whenever I liked, day or night.

We were shown the parents' area. It had a lounge with a small kitchen, four separate double bedrooms and a bathroom. Everything was new, clean and well looked after. In a few days' time, I would move to one of those rooms here for as long as it took. The rooms were available for mothers to stay the night before taking their baby home or for parents living too far to come and visit every day. We lived a two hour drive from the hospital so until she was strong enough to be transferred, I would have to stay here or come back and forth as much as possible.

The nurse came to take my catheter out. What a relief, the feeling in my legs and bum were back, and there was no pee bag hanging next to me any more.

The next day a doctor came to see me and had a list of questions for me.

How did I feel – dizzy, faint, feverish, ill?

'No, nothing.' Apart from the emotions, physically I felt absolutely fine. I could see confusion on his face. I didn't know why.

Chapter 8: Baby development facts; 23–25 weeks' gestation

The foetus/baby is thin; the body fat has not yet laid down. The skin is fragile, wrinkled and reddened. The baby loses water readily and needs to be kept warm in humid air. The genitalia are not fully developed, i.e. the boy's testicles have not descended into the scrotum and the girl's labia have not filled out so the clitoris looks prominent. The nipples are not visible yet. Tooth buds are visible under the gums. The ears look flat without lobes.

The bones are pliable. The lungs are not fully formed and if born at this age the baby will need equipment for breathing.

Most of the brain cells are in place but are not yet fully interconnected and the brain surface is smooth. Areas rich in blood vessels are particularly vulnerable to damage after birth.

The exploring movements of the early-born baby are difficult because of the effects of gravity, lack of containing support of the womb and low reserves of energy.

The taste buds are developed.

The body is sensitive to touch, particularly around the mouth. The baby demonstrates pain responses.

The hearing is well developed.

The eyes are formed although the iris lacks colour. The eyelids are still fused but are very thin and light shines through them.

A baby born this early cannot suck yet and needs to receive its feed directly into the bloodstream.

Chapter 9: 'Life in turmoil'

25th of May

I went back to see Elouisa. I would, from day one, just sit there next to her and her 'greenhouse'. I think that is a much nicer name, it was literally her little house wherein she was growing.

I would just talk to her about absolutely everything – her brothers, sister, daddy, myself, what was going on. I would tell her how well she was doing, how strong she was, and how proud we were.

That afternoon, I began feeling very weak. At first I thought it was just exhaustion after everything that had happened. I felt hot, weak, very tired and my muscles ached all over my body. I was refusing to give in and didn't want to leave Elouisa's side but had no choice, I just had to go and lie down.

I went back to my room and all I wanted to do was sleep. I asked the nurse for some painkillers. She advised the doctor that had seen me the day before. They knew this was coming.

The Healing of the 1lb Baby

The infection, strep A, the reason for the extremely premature delivery, was trying to get at me once more.

The nurse came in to take some blood, I was put on a drip with antibiotics and the nurse and doctor checked on me several times that afternoon and night.

I felt like I had fallen off the Earth; I was gone and was unaware of anything that was happening around me. I remember vaguely, only once, someone coming in to take blood. I spoke to her in Flemish, not realizing what was going on. I was delirious.

The next morning when I woke up from a seemingly very deep sleep on another planet, I felt slightly reborn.

'You really scared us there,' said a nurse. 'Happy to have you back!'

So, clearly, the doctor with all his questions had known this was coming. Months later, I would realize how dangerous my own state of health had been.

The doctor prescribed my husband and other three children antibiotics against this beast as well. It had to be eliminated completely.

26th of May

I felt like I was living in a bubble which I was not ready to come out of. Seeing Andy and the children was not possible as Orla-Jane had chickenpox and was not allowed to visit.

The third day, the nurse suggested I try to express milk. I hadn't even thought about this with the whole commotion after the birth and being unwell. Elouisa wasn't being fed yet but the milk would get frozen and used when ready.

I had always breastfed naturally. The milk always flowed freely and straight away. But this time it was very different! My breast felt as if there was nothing to give and I had to express. I felt like a cow and it hurt, it was quite a sight and

I didn't like it, especially in the beginning when nothing came out! Only after two days and by persevering, a few drops came, finally! I was ecstatic. Even though I didn't like the process, for Elouisa this milk was the best, full of antibodies and nutrients. I had to give her this.

Once the milk started, it didn't stop. I began to fill loads of bottles, which were frozen in the hospital freezer. At a certain point, I would have to take my milk home, as there was limited room in the hospital freezer and Elouisa wouldn't drink enough of it at first to make the supply go down.

I completely shut everyone out. The only person outside of Andy and the children I wanted to talk to was my sister, who had had an extremely premature baby herself. She knew what I was going through, she knew how and what I felt and nobody else did. I could not bear the thought of people reacting in sorry pitying voices calling my incredibly strong daughter 'poor...' it made me cringe, just the thought. To avoid this, I simply avoided talking to people who had never had a premature or sick baby. It was a way of protecting my positive mind – not one single fluff of negative dust was allowed in. My mind had to be one hundred per cent pure and positive, then everything would be fine. I did not want anyone to visit Elouisa. I found this completely inappropriate. She didn't look like a fresh, pink, cuddly newborn, she was a very thin, skin over bone, fighting baby. She was not an attraction. This time I was very happy to live far away from my family and far away from where we lived. It was my baby and me on our island, on our way to complete our mission. I had to heal her and she had her very first big lesson in life, to be patient and to fight like a bull, a trademark she will need in her beautiful life mission.

I received a message from my gynaecologist in Belgium. It said: 'Congratulations Marie!!!! She is a fighter, she is fantastic, trust in her, she will be fine!!! Big hugs and kisses!' She was the first person to say congratulations! The positive yellow glowing energy jumped out of my phone straight into me and filled me with strength and power. I will never ever forget this! Congratulations, indeed; the realization fell upon me: I had a baby, my fourth child was born, I had become a mother of four. Thank you.

27th of May

A whole week had passed when I was finally able to see the boys. It was a very emotional moment. We decided very consciously that the children should see their baby sister. We wanted them to understand why Mummy wasn't at home!

Adam very gently stretched out to see into the incubator. He said with his very sweet soft voice: 'She is so small.'

When they left, it hurt even more. Andy struggled with the thought that he couldn't do anything to help Elouisa or that he couldn't see her more often.

Andy's brother had passed away four years prior to this. I know that it was 'arranged' by the Universe that Andy wouldn't have to deal with this so close to that traumatic time as it would have been too much for him. I also knew that being there and dealing with this early birth was one of my life lessons. I was the one who had to learn from this. With her extremely premature birth, I would later realize, she was the most beautiful gift the Universe could have given me. I wasn't learning, trusting or believing in my healing powers so 'they' sent me Elouisa.

Almost the whole day, I would have my hands on her. I was determined. I had to heal. I knew how to give Universal energy. I just had to put my hands on her and let the Divine energy stream through me into her. I could feel my hands getting very warm. One hand on her head the other on her bum. This calmed her down within seconds. Sometimes I moved the hand from her bum to her heart as it felt needed. I knew that the Divine energy would flow to her and do the work where it was needed. When she became restless, I knew she had had enough and I left her to it.

While I had my hands on her, I closed my eyes. I imagined her lungs. Inside, the lungs are full of alveoli, little bubbles that fill with oxygen. In a baby born prematurely, the alveoli have not fully developed. Because of this and the trauma of intubation many alveoli are dead, so the lungs cannot use their full capacity to breathe properly.

I imagined a thin tube being put in her lungs, sucking out all the dead alveoli. I did this until her lungs 'looked' clear. Than I imagined her lungs being filled with the healing green colour. I waited until it felt right and I could 'see' her lungs were fully healthy, then separated the two energy systems with a (imaginary) downward movement between the two of us . This psychic surgery can also be done from a distance. When working on a person it is necessary to speak their name aloud or to use the mind.

After healing, I always feel the need to rinse my hands under streaming water just to make sure nothing has been left behind.

28th of May

Another week passed by and the lamp for jaundice was removed from Elouisa.

I could now see her fine beautiful face and long eyelashes. She tried to chew on the tube in her mouth. With the help of (a tiny piece of) glycerine tap the meconium/first poo was a reality! Funny how ecstatic a parent can be for their child to poo!

29th of May

Through her belly button, Elouisa had a 'life line', a tube through which she was given the medicine and 'food' she needed. In this way she was supplied with all the essentials she needed to live. That line had now come loose so they would have to put in another, either through the arm or leg (through one of those super-thin, tiny veins.) I found it incredibly difficult that day, watching the doctors 'fiddle' and 'hurt' her. It was too much.

They didn't manage to put in the line and eventually put in an emergency solution via her foot.

Luckily, the night team, after one and a half hours, did manage to put in a new line.

Relief!

30th of May

Andy could finally come and see her again. When she heard his voice, she wriggled and tried to open her eyes. She couldn't because they were still fused. What an amazing moment. It was beautiful to see how she reacted to his voice. It was nice to have him here. The children were at school. It was lovely to walk around outside, get some fresh air and go for a coffee.

Since her birth, Elouisa had received morphine to help her relax and to take the pain away. Exactly a week later, the morphine had been fully stopped. As a result, she was very active – more correctly, very restless. It was as if she had woken up and now fully conscious that the battle was on!

She was on the minimum intubated breathing support, which was fabulous!

Today, Elouisa received Mummy's milk for the very first time: 0.5 ml of breast milk!

She digested it well. Four hours later she got another 0.5 ml but did not digest this. The doctors decided to give her stomach a rest.

So this is how it goes, on one day there are massive highs – yes, she can do this!!! And an hour later it can slap you in the face. This is the path with an extremely prematurely born baby.

Elouisa was ten days old. I had settled in one of the parent rooms and established routine during my hospital stay. Months before, we had booked a week's holiday in France. The kids had a week off school so it would have been a lovely break before the baby came, as a few months later it would all be quite hectic again.

I told Andy to take the holiday with the children. If they were at home he would still have to keep them busy. At ten days old Elouisa was out of the 'danger zone', as we felt it, and the boys had been longing for the swimming pool holiday for a very long time.

This decision was not taken lightly. My heart was breaking at the thought of being alone, and having to carry the responsibility by myself. My heart was breaking not being able to have Andy by my side or see my children. Andy didn't want to leave me alone, what if… but we thought of the other children.

The reactions I got from certain people were painful. People judging us because my husband went on holiday while having a ten day old extremely premature baby in the NICU. I am telling you, Andy did not enjoy that trip. He would have preferred to stay at home with me, but our other three children needed this. They were desperate for Daddy's attention. They felt what was going on. Mummy wasn't there, who was normally always there, and during the week it was the grandparents looking after them, which is not the same as Mummy or Daddy. For the children, this holiday was essential. It was attention from Daddy and feeling that everything would be all right. So actually, that 'holiday' couldn't have come at a better time. No, my husband didn't leave me and our child in NICU to go on holiday, he left us to give that very important love and attention to our other children. Do not judge if you have never been in the situation yourself.

Chapter 10: Psychic surgery, closing of the duct

31st of May

The doctor explained that with such early-born babies, the duct isn't fully closed yet.

I remembered this from my sister's little boy; he ended up needing an operation to have this done. Many babies born extremely prematurely need to have their duct closed via surgery. The ductus is a small pathway between the two major blood vessels, the pulmonary artery and the aorta, leading from the baby's heart.

First the doctors try to close the duct by giving medicine. This medicine is not to be taken lightly as it could cause an intestinal perforation. It is very heavy on the heart and kidneys as well so the doctors would have to keep a very close eye on her. Why not go for the operation straight away? This procedure is, of course, even more risky on such incredibly small babies.

This problem is fairly common in premature babies.

When the baby is in the uterus it needs to have a patent

ductus as it has a completely different circulation, getting its oxygen from the placenta, to the lungs. After the baby is born, the lungs expand, the baby starts to breathe and the blood receives oxygen from the lungs. Therefore the ductus is no longer needed. The pulmonary artery is now responsible for carrying blood without oxygen away from the heart, to the lungs, where it is replenished with oxygen. The aorta is the major artery of the body and carries blood with oxygen to every part of the body. The duct that connects the two blood vessels is no longer needed. Normally the duct closes automatically when the baby is born. When a baby is born too early, the duct is not closed. The closure is necessary to help the baby to breathe by itself.

The doctor came in to make an echocardiogram of Elou-Isa's heart so they could see the open duct. I wanted to work on this with psychic surgery, in other words, fix the problem with my mind, but had no idea how to picture this. Luckily the doctor came in to explain what exactly the duct is. He explained it very visually. It is like a rugby goal, the two vertical poles being the main blood vessels, the horizontal pole that connects them the duct. When the baby is born, the horizontal connection is no longer needed. Now I knew how to visualize this, I went to my room. I said Elouisa's name out loud to make it clear who I was working on. Then I imagined in her chest the picture of the rugby goal, knowing that this was her duct. I then pictured the horizontal piece being removed and the outside wall of the big (vertical) arteries being restored. This removing of the duct with the mind can be done with imaginary knives, saws, suction... however it's done it works! I than gave what was not needed to the Angels, who carried it away to dissolve it. Do not worry about how that is done, the Universe just knows.

Once I felt it was done, I thanked every Celestial being that had helped, imagined the green colour of healing in Elouisa's chest, separated our energy systems with a downward hand movement between us and let it all go, knowing she was fine and not in need of any surgery.

The doctor gave her the medicine to close her duct. I knew she would be fine. She was not allowed any milk while receiving this medicine.

Elouisa clearly felt something was happening. She was very restless, flapping her arms around and pushing away with her hands and feet everyone that came anywhere near her. She was so small but so strong. She even managed to push her teeny tiny little bum up in the air.

Today I changed her nappy for the first time; such a small thing but so big for me. Finally I could do something for my baby.

Chapter 11:
Loneliness–oneness

1st of June

I tried to talk to her as much as possible. I explained what all the tubes were for, what the doctors and nurses were doing. I talked about the other three children, what they were doing and were going to do. I spoke about the future, what it was going to be like once she came home with us.

Today Elouisa got another glycerine tap to help her poo. It worked and I was allowed to clean her nappy and put crème on her bottom. Wonderful!

She received her second dose of medicine to close her duct. The doctors would only check for the result in a few days' time.

The infections Streptococcus A and B were under control!

Elouisa is a feisty girl!!!

2nd of June

The nurse had to increase the amount of given oxygen and give her insulin.

When born so early, the pancreas has not fully developed, which means that it cannot produce enough of the hormone insulin. This is crucially important as with not enough insulin, the body can go into shock and the baby could die as a result.

I read stories to Elouisa; it seemed to calm her down.

3rd of June

The nurse had turned down the amount of oxygen needed again. But she still gave insulin.

Elouisa had a second echocardiogram today, which showed that her duct had closed!!!! I knew this would happen. The doctor let me know that it could reopen slightly again but we would have to wait and see. I psychically checked but saw that it was definitely closed off. The doctors would later confirm this.

The fact that her duct had closed had a positive influence on her digestive system, heart and lungs. This was fantastic news.

Andy and the kiddies were in France. When I told Andy, he cried with relief.

At 15.00 one of the nurses informed me that I would have to move to another room. They needed the space for a woman who had breastfeeding problems. I finally felt like everything was settling down and I was finding 'my turn around'. I enjoyed chatting in the parents' room with those I had become friendly with, who also had had babies in the Intensive Care Unit. Now I would be moved to a building outside the hospital on my own. I was completely shaken. This might sound silly but when you are going through such an emotional situation, you feel very vulnerable. All you want and need is a bit of stability. The slightest change can throw the emotions into turmoil. I cried my eyes out, I completely blocked. I needed this routine desperately. Another couple that I was friends with were in the same position. Luckily for them, they had each other and even though they were moved to a different department, they were still in the building only a few hallways away. I tried to talk to someone but no one could do anything. This was the one thing they asked me to do and I felt as if I were falling into a deep dark hole. I felt totally alone, emotionally broken and misunderstood. The personnel did not see what this meant to me and it was the very first time since I got there that I felt absolutely, completely alone. My emotional vulnerability had filled me with fears. Even though the building was not far away, I would have to walk 'in the scary outside world that I didn't know' on my own. My mind ran away with me.

The secretary helped me with my bags. She could clearly see how distressed I was. I felt very lonely.

When I returned at the end of the day, full of emotion, I ran into two youngsters standing against the hospital wall. They were off their heads, drunk. I hung on to my handbag and was dead scared. They looked at me and started following me. They were still carrying alcohol bottles. I could hardly breathe and walked as fast as I could.

I tried to open the front door but my hands were shaking and it took ages to find the keyhole. Once I was in the building, the worst possible scenario's went through my head, my mind ran riot. In absolute fear I called the hospital being convinced I was being followed. I told the secretary that I was not staying here, I was so, so scared. I cried like a little girl. She tried to calm me down and said that security had seen them and was keeping an eye on them. These two youngsters had gone into Emergency and hadn't followed me.

I prayed to my Angels, 'Please don't let me be on my own in this building.'

Half an hour later, I heard a couple come in who were also staying in this other building. I calmed down.

I ended up enjoying my stay there, away from the hospital. It was good to just get away from everything at night.

The Healing of the 1lb Baby

What had shaken me so badly ended up being very positive.
 You are never alone but surrounded by beautiful, loving Celestial beings. Ask for help and they jump.

Chapter 12: Baby development facts; 26–28 weeks' gestation

The baby is now covered in a layer of hair called lanugo. The skin looks normal. Fat layers begin to be deposited. The sweat glands are formed but not functioning. The nipples are beginning to show. Finger and toe nails are beginning to appear but don't reach the tips yet.

A baby born at this age will need help with breathing. The digestive system is immature but small amounts of milk are given to stimulate its development.

A baby born at this gestation does not have the boundaries of the womb, which makes the body move in bursts of exaggerated jerky actions, mostly away from the body. The baby needs help to contain these movements.

The hearing is well developed and response to sound is more consistent.

The eyelids are no longer fused and the eyes open. A baby born at this gestation may show signs of distress in bright light. The eyes tend to be partly open much of the time.

Chapter 13: The healing of the energy-sucking new nurse

4th of June

Elouisa received her milk again, 0.5 ml, every hour. She digested it easily.

She was 26 weeks 'pregnancy' today!!!

5th of June

Only one day later she received 1 ml of breast milk every hour! She couldn't suck yet so the milk was given directly into her stomach.

Elouisa needed a new cannula in her foot today. The old one needed to be removed and a new one put in place.

A cannula is used to give medical personnel access to a patient's vein for the insertion of medicine or other fluids. Typically, the intravenous cannula is topped with a needle, which is used to create an opening in the body through which the tube is threaded.

While this procedure was being carried out, I stayed with her to comfort her. It was heart breaking, her whole face cried with pain but not one sound came out of her little mouth. The breathing tube pushing on the vocal cords stopped her being able to make sound. It broke my heart to see her that way but I was happy I could be there to comfort her.

The doctor decided that she needed to start breathing more independently.

Being intubated for too long could cause more harm than good as the baby would become too dependent on it. She was now put on the 'next step up' breathing support. She had to do a lot more breathing by herself.

This one was called BiPAP; Biphasic Positive Airway Pressure is a way of supporting breathing that is less invasive as the baby's airways are so tiny they can be easily damaged, which would be painful and can result in infections in the traumatized tissue. These all tubes go only a few millimetres into the baby's nostrils. BiPAP produces a constant pressure and also gives extra breaths. She didn't agree with it straight away but with the help of some more healing, she calmed down and got the hang of it by the afternoon.

I noticed today once again how magical our connection is. I feel at one with this child, I feel connected in the deepest part of my soul.

She opened her eyes. She tried so hard! It asked tons of energy to open her eyes but she did it. It was her way of showing her response to me. She reacted very much to my voice.

What a strong little girl. We are so proud. I found out today, without knowing this beforehand, that Elouisa means 'Famous warrior'. What an incredible person she is.

I missed Andy, Jack, Adam and Orla-Jane.

6th of June

I walked in to see Elouisa. One of the nurses introduced me to a new, trainee nurse. She had come from another hospital to gain further experience on this ward.

The second I laid eyes on her, I felt very uncomfortable. Something did not feel right. I put this feeling to one side because I didn't want to judge her; how could I think this not even knowing this person? It would come to the surface very quickly, though, that I wasn't judging, but following my gut feeling.

That day, every baby in its incubator in that room had some difficulty. Every baby had constant saturation dropping, 'forgot' to breathe, was nervous, restless and unsettled. Doctors and nurses were saying all around me: 'What is going on today!'

Then I saw energetically what was happening, that 'the new nurse' was literally sucking the fighting spirit energy away from the babies to herself. She was the type of person, so down on herself, lacking confidence, that she was sucking other people's energy to keep herself happy. She was desperately looking for youth and strength. A place like the NICU is full of fighting, battling, incredibly strong energies! She would also just sit with the babies with her hands on them. No other nurse would do this. They did their job; looked after them, treated them, but did not do what mothers did, sit with them for ages with their hands on the babies. It was unbearable. Even though I didn't fancy doing healing on this because I had enough on my plate, again, there was a reason why she was there while I was there. This had to stop, especially as this lady was working on an NICU ward! She would do more harm than good! So I went into my room and imagined the ward. I imagined big pipes in each corner of the room and saw how all these energies from her were sucked out of the room. Then I placed her in a big balloon-like circle with green healing light in it. Around every child's incubator, I imagined a big bright circle of light as protection. This way, negative energies couldn't penetrate. In the coming days, I would do this every morning and every evening. I could feel during the day how angrily she reacted towards me. There were aggressive feelings. I found all this quite scary! I called Carine, my spiritual friend, to ask for confirmation and advice on this. Carine confirmed what I saw was happening and the reason why this nurse reacted so aggressively towards me was because (of course, unconsciously) she felt I was trying to stop her. As a result, she was desperate, like a drug addict, to get to the positive energies she was seeking! One moment when I had just finished washing my hands, she came and literally pushed me aside. I was shocked. The anger coming out of that push was enormous!

After all the work I did, I did not see her sit with the babies any more and she never sat with Elouisa. I had asked the Universe to keep her away from Elouisa and she stayed away.

All the healing and protecting was doing its work, and by the second week everything had calmed down. I thought it never would. By the time 'the work was done', she left. I was shattered!

The spiritual doctor (I will talk about her later on) asked me if I was OK. I told her there had been someone sucking energy from the babies and spreading unpleasant energies.

'I know, it was that trainee nurse, I saw it,' she said.

That was another confirmation. And I had learned a new lesson and had a beautiful healing under my belt.

From that day on I liked imagining a bright circle of light around Elouisa's incubator so no negative energies could enter and she would have the time to get her physical body growing and strong. Next to her I placed a big strong Angel, like a bouncer. I could see him standing next to her with his arms crossed, shining with light. I am telling you, anyone with negative energy would run a mile and not come anywhere near her!

7th of June

With such a premature baby it happens a lot that the baby 'forgets to breathe'. It is very upsetting to see for the parent. Suddenly the baby goes all floppy like a ragdoll and grey. It is literally as the soul leaves the body. The nurse taps the bottom firmly, sits the baby up and rubs the feet. Just any stimulation possible is tried to get the baby to breathe again. It happens, as it did with Elouisa; that the nurse needs to apply 'bagging'. She then pumps air into her lungs with a medical 'bag' and increases the oxygen supply.

I found it difficult to watch this when it happened. I knew it was 'normal' for this to happen, but easy, no.

She's been weighed: 626 grams! After she was born, like every newborn, her weight had gone down, to 480 grams. Two weeks later being at 626 grams was a fabulous moment!

8th of June

Her breathing went so much better today.

The nurse looking after her was changing her linen. He asked me if I wanted to help. 'Yes, please, what can I do?' I asked. 'You can lift her,' he said. I stood there with my mouth open – wow, I could 'hold' her. All I had done since she was born was put my hands on her. This was the closest I had been to her since she was born. This was the most beautiful experience. It was a fabulous feeling to feel her body weight. She fitted snuggly in my hands, my tiny little baby. I felt emotional and she was very relaxed. This was THE high point of the day; no, of the last two weeks!

Chapter 14: Psychic surgery, go away bug

9th of June

I arrived this morning and Elouisa had had difficulty overnight with breathing. They took a blood sample and sent it to the lab. The reason was that a 'bug' was growing, a virus. They didn't know yet what exactly. The funny thing was that even though she stopped breathing more often and it concerned the doctors, when they checked the oxygen levels in her blood, there was no problem at all. No stress!

It was scary when she 'stopped' breathing and also her heart rate dropped.

The doctors were cautious and gave her antibiotics. I gave her healing.

I felt down today. I was worried. Just for a moment, negative thinking tried to enter my mind. I waved it away and went to my room.

I said Elouisa's name out loud. I saw little creatures in her body. I put an imaginary tube through her skin into her blood and sucked all of the creatures out until there were none left. Beautiful Celestial beings caught them in a bag and carried them away from her to be dissolved. I imagined now that her blood was flowing healthily. I could see her glowing. I trusted more and more. I started to realize this technique really works.

We are from nature perfectly healthy. When we get ill, it is because something has become too heavy in our mind. It is a way of showing, 'I have it difficult with something'. This was the same case with Elouisa. She was, by getting ill from a virus, clearly showing that she found things hard. She was not happy and was tired. She got tired of the prodding and pulling. She got tired of the constant hard work to stay in that tiny little body. I went back to her and spoke to her. 'I know it is hard, darling, I know it is awful constantly having needles put in your legs and arms, I know it is so hard having to breathe with your so small body. No, you know what, I don't know, but I can imagine. But listen, Elouisa, you are doing so well, you are so incredibly strong, we are so, so proud of you. Every day it will become easier. Every day you get stronger and one day this will all be over and you will be playing with your brothers and sister. You will be cuddling with Mummy and Daddy. You will be laughing with Orla-Jane. You will be running after them, having fun and being their little bug. This is only now. This will pass, quicker than you think. You are a fighter. You are doing so well. I love you so, so much.'

10th of June

She had a very good night but by 8.30 all of a sudden the medical staff had decided to put her back on the full intubation. Apparently this happens quite often. They said she was exhausted. Her right lung was collapsing. Being back on the full intubation was purely to let her rest and come back to strength. I had to trust.

Elouisa received another blood transfusion. This happens because such small babies don't renew their red blood cells quickly. Because they are born early, preemies may develop a type of anaemia called anaemia of prematurity. In the last weeks of pregnancy, two changes occur that help full term babies to make red blood cells. First, a lot of the iron needed to make new red blood cells is transferred from the mother to the baby in the third trimester. Also, in the last weeks of pregnancy, red blood cell production switches from the liver to the bone marrow. Because the processes that make new red blood cells are immature in preemies, preemies have a higher rate of anaemia and their anaemia is more severe than in term babies. NICU care can make anaemia in preterm infants worse. Doctors and nurses try to limit the amount of blood that's drawn for lab tests, but even small blood losses can affect very small preemies. After receiving blood, it is magical how life 'returns' in them and they are suddenly doing so well.

I did some more healing. I imagined her lung, put some healing reiki symbols in her right lung and opened it up with my mind until I saw a healthy beautiful lung. I checked the left one as well. Then I filled them up with the green healing colour to keep the healing going. Seeing that it was her right lung, it meant it was connected to her father's side. I gave all Andy's worries back to him, away from her. I put some healing reiki symbols on the father–daughter connection and gave them each their own energy field with a downward hand movement between the two of them. Then I did the same between me and her so everyone had their own energy system. I felt peace.

11th of June

The doctors never found the virus, they thought something was 'growing' but nothing was ever found. So it went as quickly as it came. This was no coincidence. I started to trust deeply – our mind is so strong!!! It all happens up there!

The doctor said how well she was doing. This meant so much to me because the doctors are very careful with their words. They don't just give 'compliments'. This made my day.

12th June

What a fabulous day.

The doctors started to talk about transfer in two to four weeks. Elouisa looked really good and was back on minimum breathing support. The doctor said again how happy he was with her progress!

The antibiotics were stopped as there was no infection or bacteria.

In the afternoon she went back to the BiPAP! Breathing more independently! I felt so happy, another step forward. At the same time I held my breath. My beautiful darling, only positive thoughts, only positive thoughts, our natural state is perfect health.

Chapter 15: Guilt towards the other children

13th of June

Elouisa was receiving more milk, 2 ml every hour, and digesting it very well!

She still had moments where she suddenly stopped breathing and where her heart rate just dropped. When that happened, my heart stopped.

This day, every time I came closer, holding her, touching her, she stopped breathing and became very restless. I was all over the place, desperately wanting to be with her. I had this overwhelming feeling and desperation that I needed to heal her. I could not leave. I had to be there all the time, because what if suddenly something happened and I wasn't there to heal! I had noticed so clearly what a fabulous job the healing was doing, how with the mind and Universal energy energies were being lifted, changed for the better, so she could return to her natural state of perfect health and that I should now not let go. This was clearly the next step in my lesson – to trust! Elouisa was telling me through all her anxiousness, the breath stoppage and heart rate drop that I had to leave her alone. It had become too much. She now needed some time to take over and heal herself. I had learnt and done an enormous job but now she needed some space.

I felt that I was ignoring this big message from above. I felt it, I knew it!

There was a clear reason why exactly that day I received a phone call from Carine.

I wasn't listening to my guides and Angels so 'they' tried a new route. 'Out of the blue' Carine started talking about this whole subject I had met and was ignoring! As she said, having such a strong mother 'taking over' to keep going and going and going, my daughter needed her turn now; I had to trust my daughter.

Also this exact same day I received a phone call from my friend who had been looking after the other children the past week. I had been ignoring the feeling of how terribly I missed them as a protection for myself. I was torn in two directions. I couldn't leave Elouisa. What if she gave up because she didn't know where Mummy was? What if Elouisa thought I didn't love her any more and had left her? The other direction was my other three fabulous children, who were missing me terribly.

My friend was really good with the kids. I know her well, she listens and talks to the children and is very much in touch with their emotions. The kids felt comfortable and open with her. I already knew that. I had asked her to come to England and look after them, to take over from the grandparents for a bit.

She told me that, a few nights ago, my eldest son Jack was watching the TV. He sat there tired and alone, his shoulders and arms just hanging down. She noticed this and said, 'Jack, are you okay?' Jack didn't move and cried non-stop. All the emotions of the last month came out. He had had fights with his granddad and he missed me terribly to talk to. He missed Mummy so much. My friend said that Jack cried for at least ten minutes, shoulders shaking, sitting there like a miserable heap of sadness.

When she was dropped off at the grandparents' or nursery, Orla-Jane screamed her lungs out.

Adam, as always, kept everything inside. He just came closer to my friend to ask for cuddles, which he does rarely.

This message on top of the phone call with Carine and my own message from above that I had now accepted made me decide it was time to go home.

Suddenly I felt ready. The bubble popped. I accepted this and was actually looking forward to going home. Organized as I am I needed a plan. So the plan was that I would go home for two nights and than go back again to stay with Elouisa. It would take pressure off Andy and the grandparents and everyone would be able to settle a bit. This way, I could be there for all four of my children. In a few days' time, Andy would pick me up.

Elouisa was three weeks old today.

Chapter 16: The spiritual Healing doctor

14th of June

Elouisa lost some weight; down to 590 grams. Her weight was an obsession!

The whole change of breathing support and the stopping of milk for a few days had caused this.

The experience from the day before had calmed me down. The fact that I had accepted the message and 'backed off' had calmed Elouisa down. This day I was given a challenge straight away. It was as if they were saying above 'let's see if she has really taken on the message'.

As Elouisa grew stronger in her little greenhouse, I would sit next to her to do some studying. One of the doctors showed an interest in what I was reading. She said, 'Do you study art?'

'No, I'm learning about the working of Crystals,' I said.

I was a bit shy to tell her this, a scientific person would probably be very sceptical about that type of healing, but, hey, she asked me so I wasn't going to lie.

'Fantastic!' she said, 'I am very interested in the spiritual healing world as well.'

I couldn't believe it. A doctor who is interested in spiritual healing!

After that 'meeting', more often she would come and sit next to me to talk. We would have some very interesting conversations over the next few weeks.

She told me, she had had enough of the medical rules and regulations, the whole scientific world. She was longing to do more healing the natural way.

She could also see the premature babies 'fly' between earthly life and spirit at the beginning of their lives. She had also witnessed how Elouisa went back and forth from her body to spirit during the first ten days of her life. This is the time when these souls make the decision to stay or go back. If they choose to go back, they might come back to Earth later, in another pregnancy/another body. I sometimes saw this lady with her hands gently above the babies, only briefly. Now I knew she was giving them beautiful Universal energy. At that point she didn't realize how important it was her being there, what a fabulous job she was doing with these babies.

One evening I looked in the cards, interested to see who she was. She was a very spiritually powerful woman and her cards and energy were incredible! She still had a long learning path to travel as she would have to learn to channel that energy. Sometimes I wonder what she is doing now...

Elouisa had been off the full intubation for several days. Her saturations kept dropping and the doctors suggested to intubate her again. They said it was normal, that it happens sometimes. This would only be for a day or so, to give her another rest. She was exhausted having to breathe partially on her own. This would revive her strength. Even though I was disappointed and saw this as a step back, what could

I do? And I had promised to let her find her own healing strength!

The spiritual doctor was there that day and would do the procedure. They asked me to wait in the parents' room while this was happening. It would only take five minutes. I ended up waiting there for at least half an hour. But I was a good girl, didn't do any healing and waited.

The spiritual doctor came in after ten minutes to tell me to hang on. After another ten minutes, she came in again to tell me to be patient, always with a relaxing smile on her face. I was wondering what was going on!

Eventually she came back with the news that they did not have to intubate her. The spiritual doctor told me she 'knew', she 'felt', that Elouisa did not need to go back to full intubation. This was purely her gut feel as you could call it. She was receiving this information from Higher up, it is a knowing. The big thing was, of course, how long she could prolong this waiting before she made a decision wether or not to intubate? Because, OK, she knew Elouisa could do it without full intubation, but how long could she wait responsibly? How long could she justify this waiting, medically? I fully understood her. And I know she would never ever push it to the limit! Just before the point that she couldn't wait any longer medically, she said to Elouisa: 'Come on, girl, I know you can do it, show us, otherwise I will have to intubate you again!'

Elouisa's saturations went up again and stayed stable long enough to show the doctors she was fine.

My dear spiritual doctor, you are doing Angel work!

The Universe has its healers 'hidden' and placed everywhere. How beautifully it works!

I felt so proud of myself and Elouisa. I had not sabotaged, ignored or disbelieved but listened to the Universal message, I had trusted their message and I had trusted and believed in my daughter. Look what a result you then get: beautiful healing and luck. Everything is in Divine right order. 'They' do know best.

15th of June

Overnight Elouisa had received another blood transfusion. She looked radiant again! Wonder blood! The nurse involved me in absolutely everything. Today we were having a first small cuddle. Not the real full-on cuddle. For that her breathing hadn't been stable enough. The nurse took her out on the mattress and laid her on my lap. It was magical to see my tiny little baby (she still looked incredibly small) from so close with no plastic from the incubator between us. She looked so petite, tiny, lovely, fine, and absolutely perfect.

During the day I was allowed to 'lift' her several times while the nurse changed her sheets or sit her up while something else was done. It was just incredible to feel her little body.

The nurse took off Elouisa's hat and for the very first time I was able to see her full head. She had black hair and was, in my eyes, absolutely beautiful. The nurse even took off her breathing mask for a few seconds while I took a picture. She was very relaxed and just kept breathing nicely.

The nurse showed me how to massage her body with oil. Elouisa absolutely loved this. She was awake a lot today and very alert. She was looking around with big open eyes and than gave me her very first smile! This is love, this is what real love feels like.

16th of June

We had our first kangaroo-cuddle!!!!!

My baby was three weeks old and I finally got to hold her properly, skin on skin! What a moment. What a palaver though to hold my baby. Two people helping to get all the tubes and wires in the correct place and place her on my chest. But that moment when skin touched skin, I was lost for words. Everything fell into place.

'Are you okay?' said the nurse.

I smiled and cried 'Yes'.

This we had been waiting for, my little girl.
It was magical.
Everything around me stopped.
My ears did not hear any more, my eyes only saw this tiny little girl.
All I did was enjoy.
I consciously let her feel my breathing.
We were one again.

Chapter 17: Adjustment to the outside world

17th of June

Today Andy came with the children to pick me up to go home for the first time since I had arrived in hospital, still pregnant.

I went downstairs to the hospital hall to wait for them. My heart was beating like mad. I was nervous. I was shivering from excitement. It was busy in the hall. I was early. When I finally saw Andy holding Orla-Jane's hand, walking through that door, I burst into tears. She suddenly looked so big. The boys were chatting away. I cried when I hugged Orla-Jane, who was very confused and clinging on to Andy. Jack, open as always, swung himself around me. Adam just stood there not knowing what to do with himself until I picked him up and gave him the biggest cuddle ever. I was so excited to go home, to take a breather. We spent the day at the seaside, a lovely day with the family. In the back of my mind, Elouisa.

As we drove further and further away, it was as if my heart was being pulled out. This feeling would be the same when I went back to the hospital, I would find it very hard to leave home. All I wanted now was for our baby to come home but we weren't there just yet.

It was quite an adjustment coming back into 'the real world'. Everyone felt rude, hard, rushing and insensitive to me. I had felt so strong and positive in hospital but when I came out, I couldn't cope with all the impressions from the outside world.

As I walked outside, seeing mums with prams and newborn babies, I wanted to shout that I had a baby too! I wanted to tell everyone that I had an 'after pregnancy body' because I had just had a baby.

It felt as if everyone was looking at me wondering where my baby was.

I would feel so proud going to the supermarket buying a pack of nappies to take to the hospital because then people would see that I had a baby. I wanted the whole world to see me with a pack of nappies! I had to buy the smallest nappies and Elouisa would fit in them completely. That would be a few weeks on.

I loved just mooching around baby clothes shops. This was still very premature and even though I ended up buying the smallest clothes ever on specialized premature baby websites it felt so nice to 'belong to the newborn baby mums'. I would get this satisfaction by walking through baby clothes shops. I would end up buying a nice blanket, wash it at sixty degrees and than wrap it up so no germs could get to it to take it to the hospital. Or a little bear that wasn't even allowed in her incubator.

Dealing with everyone's questions was the hardest of all. Not everyone knows how to react. Do we talk or do we leave her alone? So they end up staring or whispering. I can imagine that no one meant harm, but it was hard to deal with. The staying positive in my mind was also hard now I had to share facts with other people. I couldn't avoid the 'poor...' any more.

I had a new lesson. Give their reactions back to them and let it go. They meant well.

One day I took the boys to school. I heard one of the mums whisper behind me, 'Oh my God, that's that woman with that baby!' I felt so angry and wanted to turn around and shout that 'that baby' was stronger than her and any other person walking around there. My protective mother instinct was enormous, ready to go into battle for every whisper, word or bad thought. Feeling this way made me very tired.

It would get easier.

Elouisa was at 28 weeks 'pregnancy' today.

Chapter 18: Baby development facts: 28–30 weeks' gestation

The baby is beginning to put on fat and doesn't look so thin and wrinkled any more. The fingernails are formed. The lanugo (hair on the body) is thinning and is likely to be most noticeable on the shoulders. The nipples are visible but are flat and pale.

If born now, some babies can manage breathing without breathing support.

The brain is going through a rapid growth and development with millions of connections being made between cells. Its development is influenced by experience, whether in or outside the uterus. The folds that differentiate different functional areas of the brain are more visible.

A baby born at this age will still have exaggerated movements. The baby does make efforts to self calm.

The eyes can open and close. If the baby is born at this age, they will be most able to open their eyes in the shade.

True sleep patterns emerge but sleep is mainly light with rapid eye movements.

The newborn baby may suck its thumb or fingers for comfort.

Chapter 19: Not just for me; healing of a full term baby with life threatening lung problems

Walking back and forth day after day from the NICU to my room, I felt this heavy energy around a baby boy lying there. He had been in distress during birth and had defecated in the water and started breathing it in while still in the womb. This had damaged his lungs and potentially also his brain. He had been intubated and was still on the NICU with breathing help and severe problems. Having enough on my plate already with my own baby, I tried to ignore all the other things I was feeling. Clearly, the Universe thought differently about this and wanted me to learn, heal and trust!

I couldn't ignore this any longer. My big question towards the Universe was first: 'Am I allowed to heal without someone's permission?'

The answer from above was: 'You can only do good with healing from the heart, which you are doing. Heal, and then it is up to them to receive or reject it. This is the free will of human beings. If you were not allowed to heal it, it wouldn't cross your path.'

I sat down in my room and pictured that baby boy in my mind. I used psychic surgery to fully cleanse his lungs of meconium and damaged cells.

I would imagine all the 'bad things' being sucked out of his lungs and carried away by Angels to be dissolved, until his lungs were cleared. I would picture little tubes going in his lungs that would drain away the 'bad things'. Once his lungs looked clear, I would picture his lungs filled with a beautiful green colour. Green is a healing colour.

As I asked (the Universe) if there was anything else, it was made clear to me that a family circle coming from the father's side was at the base of this problem.

I want to press on every reader's heart that guilt is not ever what we want to feel here! This all happens unconsciously and there is nothing you can do about this, except to work on yourself and heal your energy system when ready to do so.

I could see a blanket of emotional problems now lying on the child coming from the father. With the help of Universal energy I moved all of that energy away from the baby back to the father. I pictured it being moved from him to his father. I could see energetically that the father started crying heavily as he got his 'package' back. The child lit up and was shining, clearly very happy with these burdened energies taken away.

It was too heavy for the father to carry and I could already see it came from his mother, so I helped him to energetically give it back to her. Whatever was left with him I surrounded with a healing green colour so he would heal this and did the same with his mother.

I later heard from the baby's mother, whom I met regularly in the parents' room, that her baby boy was progressing well and the doctors were hopeful. They had to wait for a brain scan to know if any damage had occurred to his brain. I could feel he would be fine.

Chapter 20: A baby on the ward passes away

A baby boy had been brought to the ward. He was in the second half of the room. I didn't see him but knew what was going on. I understood he was a newborn. His mum had fallen asleep with him in her arms. When she woke up he looked blue. No one knew what had happened. When he arrived at the hospital they said he had already 'gone' but they kept his body alive with machinery so the family could say a proper goodbye. They bathed him, cuddled him and spoke to him. The mother's parents stayed in one of the parents' rooms on the ward. They had the room next to mine.

The next day they turned off the machines and the little boy passed away. The sadness felt on the ward was enormous. Screens were set up around the baby and nurses were trying to comfort the parents and family.

I had a 'look' to make sure the baby boy went to the Light but he had already gone. I was told his spirit had already returned when they arrived at the hospital the day before.

The next day after they left, one of the sisters asked me to change rooms. They needed my room for someone else. She asked me to take the room next door. As you probably can guess, it was the room where the grandparents of the baby boy had stayed. Even though the new person could have gone in that room, they wanted me to move into it. It didn't make any sense whatsoever, but I could guess the reason. The Universe wanted me in that room to heal the energies. I entered that room and I could hardly stand in it. The energy fell on me like a big heavy block, I almost started crying. It was highly unpleasant. It was not the place to sleep in while having to be strong with a baby in a high dependency unit! So, there you go! I was starting to understand my mission.

I went into the toilet to do the healing. I could not do it sitting in that room, it just felt too heavy. In the toilet I wouldn't be disturbed...

I imagined the room and put in four pipes, one in each corner, to let the sad, heavy energies leave the room. I placed reiki symbols of healing and insight in the room and saw how everything cleared up. At the end, I separated my own energy from that of the room with a downward hand movement between the room and myself, using my imagination.

Once I was back in the room I asked my Angels to protect my aura from these energies and I placed a Clear Quartz and an Amethyst in the room. I luckily had a box of Crystals with me.

Clear Quartz is pure healing, the purest light that dispels all darkness. Amethyst purifies any energies that need purifying and gives calmness.

I left the room to let everything do its work. When I returned a few hours later, the room had been cleansed of previous energies.

Chapter 21: Swollen tummy and water retention

20th of June

Elouisa was now receiving 5 ml of milk every hour and weighed 660 grams!

I hadn't seen her for two days and she looked like she had grown. The two days that I was away she had done really well and had hardly stopped breathing. The break from 'full-on mummy' had done her good. It had done me the world of good also to go away. As I said, the outside world was hard, but being in my home with Andy and the children had been good for the soul.

The number of impulses given by the BiPAP had been reduced.

We had an hour cuddle. Heaven!

23rd of June

29 weeks' 'pregnancy'!

Elouisa had received since the day before extra powdered

milk in my breast milk to increase the calorie intake. She was still being fed directly into the stomach.

24th of June
I went home again and this time I wished I hadn't left.
I was allowed to call the hospital as often as I wanted. When I called, a nurse always came on the phone to answer my questions or just tell to me how Elouisa's day had been.
This day she wasn't very well.
Her tummy was swollen and hard. Her heart rate kept dropping and she needed a lot of extra oxygen again. The feeds had to be stopped again. Maybe it was the added powdered milk that had caused this.
We knew that moments like this were going to happen.
I was worried. It was Andy who reminded me to trust.
I took a deep breath while looking out of the window into the outstretched landscape. As I relaxed I could feel the answer about my worry. I was worrying for nothing. She would be fine.

26th of June
And, indeed, two days later she was a lot better. They started feeding again, without the added powdered milk, and slowly but surely, the administered oxygen had been turned down.
The hard swollen tummy had gone. She was now swollen around the groin and legs. This was water retention. This is a result of the heart having to work so hard and not pumping efficiently; it is a form of heart failure, which in preterm infants is treatable, unlike in an old person with a damaged and diseased heart. She was given diuretics for this.

28th of June
I went back to the hospital after having been home for a few days.
I was so excited to see her again. I started to really feel

the benefit of going home. I had stopped waking up in the middle of the night to express milk. I had a massive supply of breast milk in the freezer and wanted to catch up on sleep. I remembered very well how it is with a baby at home at night! I really had enough of all that 'pumping' and somewhere I felt that I wouldn't go on to the actual breastfeeding once Elouisa was ready. I found those bottles a lot less tiring!

Her head looked bigger today, funny how you notice every little change.

She was receiving powdered milk/fortifier in her milk again and digested it beautifully.

29th of June

As Elouisa grew steadily, I was enjoying her. Nappy changing, talking to her, cuddles and massage with baby oil. It calmed her down immediately.

She weighed 718 grams!

Elouisa's breathing support had changed again to the next step up. Fantastic! This one was called CPAP; Continuous Positive Airway Pressure is a way of supporting breathing that is the same as BiPAP apart from one big difference, and step forward: no extra breaths are given.

2nd of July

Slowly but surely, many of my 'NICU mummy buddies' were starting to be transferred to hospitals closer to home. Well, the babies were. Somehow, even though Elouisa was still so little, I felt like I could see the light at the end of the tunnel. It seemed like there was a shift in people. The mums I had shared many hours with, who had been so supportive, all seemed to be leaving; starting the next step in their story.

Everything was changing. I felt like I became less attached to the hospital. I was happy to walk outside, laughing again with people who were close to me.

Elouisa was at 30 weeks' 'pregnancy'.

3rd of July

Elouisa weighed 750 grams!

When I arrived at the hospital the nurse gave me a fabulous picture of Elouisa.

Something so 'silly' means the world to a mum with a baby in the Intensive Care Unit. The fact that the nurse took the time and thought to take a picture for me made my day.

This same day, Elouisa had come off the CPAP for a whole hour! I couldn't have been more proud. Another push forward.

4th of July

Elouisa was six weeks old today!!!

7th of July

I had only been at home for two days and I missed her so much. This time I stayed at home and Andy went and stayed over for one night. It went completely against my mother instinct. This ripped my heart out. It was a weekend of floods of tears. All I wanted was to be with my baby.

She was weighed and was now 865 grams. The fortifier added to my milk was doing her good.

Chapter 22: Baby development facts; 31–33 weeks' gestation

The eyelashes and eyebrows are well developed. The baby is beginning to fill out and looks plumper. The fingernails have now grown to the finger tips.

The digestive system may be mature enough to tolerate full milk feeding. Breast milk is more likely to be tolerated than formula. Very often with extremely premature babies, fortifier/formula will be added to breast milk to raise the calorie content.

The lungs may be mature enough for the baby to breathe on his own if born at this age, although some extra oxygen may be needed and some babies need mechanical assistance.

The brain is growing fast and creases that separate the different lobes are obvious. From now on the front part of the brain goes through a major growth spurt.

A baby born at this age tends to have sudden, big, jerky outward movements of the legs and arms but is more able to tuck limbs in.

The baby will make efforts to pay attention to a voice or

soft sound or a face provided the surroundings are quiet and softly lit and the stimulus is presented gently.

The eye is growing rapidly and is vulnerable to damage arising from the physiological instability. When born at this age, a baby may also look at and follow an object in quiet, subdued lighting. Eye movements are not well coordinated.

The baby is now capable of sleeping deeply as well as lightly.

Chapter 23:
Eyes and ears

11th of July

Elouisa was seven weeks old.

Slowly but surely, the doctors were weaning her off the CPAP. The CPAP produces a constant pressure at the nose that is transmitted to the lungs. The newly introduced next level up breathing support only gives her a constant low flow of extra oxygen via a nasal cannula.

This day she was two hours on light constant oxygen flow and eight hours on the CPAP. The CPAP hours will be steadily decreased until she is completely weaned off. This is the last step before breathing without breathing support.

15th of July

She weighed 975 grams! That one kilo was smiling at us! What an obsession with the weight of a preemie.

A hospital closer to home had accepted Elouisa. This meant that she would be transferred by ambulance to another hospital. When the doctor first told me, I had a double feeling. On one hand ecstatic, on the other very scared. We were so used to this hospital, the staff... We had full trust in every person working there. I knew that this transfer was a good sign. It meant she was doing so well that she was strong enough to be transferred and a smaller hospital would be able to look after her. This was good!

The transfer would now depend on the schedule of the ambulance and her.

16th–19th of July

Elouisa was retaining a lot of fluid again, which meant that breathing on normal flow oxygen was made difficult. These four days, the doctors felt it was better for her to stay on the CPAP. When retaining fluid, the alveoli are moist as well, which made it a lot harder to breathe.

Elouisa received her first immunization. She reacted absolutely fine, no reactions just very tired.

Today she had her second eye test.

In the womb the eyes start to develop at about sixteen weeks. The most rapid growth and development occurs during the last twelve weeks of pregnancy.

Experts think that premature birth interrupts the eye growth, which can lead to ROP (retinopathy of prematurity).

Premature babies are at risk for ROP because the retina (the membrane at the back of the eye that helps transform light into images) is less developed and only partially covered with blood vessels at birth. Many premature babies get supplemental oxygen soon after birth. High levels of oxygen, or fluctuation in a baby's oxygen level, can damage the partially formed blood vessels of the retina.

ROP causes blood vessels in the eye to grow abnormally and spread throughout the retina. These new blood vessels are fragile and leak blood into the eye. Scar tissue can form and pull the retina away from the back of the eye, causing vision loss. It usually affects both eyes and is the leading cause of vision loss in children. Babies who are born weighing about 2¾ lbs or less and are born earlier than 32 weeks/

The Healing of the 1lb Baby

especially before 28 weeks are at the highest risk for retinopathy of prematurity. It can be treated and many babies' eyesight has been 'saved' thanks to early finding and laser treatment.

A few weeks earlier, when this first came up, I started healing on Elouisa's eyes before the check-up. I wanted to be sure I had done this before the doctor came. I would place my hand on her eyes, also covering her Third Eye. The Third Eye is situated between the eyebrows. Eye problems have their energetic place in the Third Eye. When there are problems with the eyes, it means that there is a blockage in the Third Eye. This energy point can get blocked by the following:

- What you see is not always synonymous with what you've been told
- Invalidation of intuitive and psychic experiences
- Ugly or frightening environment (war, violence)

Because in this case we are talking about premature babies, these events could have their roots in past lives and cause a Third Eye blockage.

I would lay my hand on Elouisa's eyes and ask the Universe to let healing energy stream through me into her eyes. I could feel and see the energy coming in through the top of my head – my Crown chakra – streaming through my body and coming out of my hands into Elouisa's eyes. I would keep this up until it felt enough. I would repeat this several times as long as it felt needed. I also placed reiki healing and strength symbols in her eyes and the Insight and Healing reiki symbol on her Third Eye. I would see fine impurities coming out of her eyes as they were being healed. I waved them away from her eyes as they were coming out to be taken away to be purified by Celestial beings. I trusted and knew that her eyes were fine. The first eye test confirmed this and the second made it completely clear that her eyes were in perfect condition. She was in no need of laser treatment.

Her ears had been tested as well.
Premature babies are at increased risk for hearing abnormalities and should have their hearing tested before discharge from the hospital. If the tests are abnormal, the baby should see a specialist for further evaluation and treatment.
The doctor had noticed some fluid in one of her ears. Nothing worrying, but she would have to be followed up once home.

She was 32 weeks 'pregnancy' and weighed 1.030 kg!!! Hooray!!!
She also received another blood transfusion. I always liked this because I knew how much energy it would give her.

I was at home when the hospital called me to say that the ambulance was there to pick Elouisa up and transfer her to the other hospital. This transfer is quite the thing. The baby is put into a different incubator. It takes ages to 'rewire' everything and make sure everything the baby needs is connected and working well. I had seen it several times while being in hospital with her. We were there a while, several people came and went. Now it was our turn!
After the phone call, I didn't know what to do with myself. She would be going back to the hospital that I was first admitted to just before she was born. I felt very nervous. No more two hours' driving to go and see my little girl, no more leaving of the family or having to depend on other people to look after my other children. Normal life would finally return. But I felt very anxious as something wasn't right.
Two hours later I had another phone call. Elouisa had not been transferred. After half an hour on the journey, her

oxygen levels kept dropping and the accompanying nurse didn't feel comfortable, not even being half way to the hospital.

I think Elouisa had freaked out. No one had spoken to her about what was about to happen and I wasn't there to do that. It was her way of saying 'Hang on, I don't know where I'm going, I don't like this!'

Later I would also notice that I would have to be in another, different, hospital for healing work. We weren't meant to go back to where we had been before she was born.

So there you go, a few more two-hour trips would have to be made, but to be honest, I didn't mind. Once Elouisa was back in the hospital she didn't have any more saturation dropping and was absolutely fine and a contented little madam.

25th of July

Elouisa was now able to breathe four hours on normal oxygen flow and than alternately four hours on the CPAP.

She was nine weeks old, at 33 weeks' pregnancy and weighed 1.258 kg!

30th of July

We were at 34 weeks' 'pregnancy', 10 weeks old and weighing 1.435 kg!

Elouisa was now five hours without and three hours with CPAP. It was going in favour of normal oxygen flow.

Oh, I was so longing to have her with us at home.

1st of August

What a day. After a whole month of weaning, she was fully off the CPAP!!! Elouisa was now breathing on her own receiving a very small but constant amount of oxygen via a nasal cannula. No more impulses to remind her to breathe, she was doing that by herself. She would still forget sometimes but, hey, she was still in hospital being kept an eye on and was still six weeks away from being 'born' so we were not going to fall out over that futility.

3rd of August

She was moved away from Intensive Care to the Special Care Unit. This was a big moment. My little girl in a normal baby (hospital) bed. She had several layers of clothes on, wrapped up under big, warm, soft blankets. Only her little head was peeping out from underneath. The nurse had to keep a close eye on her temperature. She had no more incubator to keep her warm, her greenhouse was gone, she had to do this by herself.

Chapter 24: Transfer closer to home

6th of August

Elouisa had finally been transferred!

She ended up in another hospital than originally asked for as that one was now full. I already felt there would be work to do in this hospital. It would be the third hospital I had been to since my waters broke.

Before she was transferred, I had spoken to Elouisa and explained what was going to happen. I told her not to panic when the nurses moved her into an incubator and she was driven away in an ambulance. I told her the trip was a good thing because it meant she was coming closer to home and I would be there once she got there and was settled. I heard afterwards that the trip had gone smoothly. Elouisa had had no saturation drops and had been relaxed.

I had read about this hospital and it had had many unpleasant happenings in the past. My initial feeling wasn't very good and I was the least excited that my daughter had ended up there. What could I do? I knew there would be a healing job to be done.

After ten weeks in Intensive Care, my little darling was now only a short trip away in a Special Care Unit.

The hospital rang me to tell me that she had arrived well and I was more than welcome to come and see her.

When I arrived at the parking, I stayed in the car for ten minutes. It was not too busy and I had a full view of the hospital.

Before I went in I wanted to cleanse the energies. So I placed (imagined) big pipes on each corner of the hospital, going into the ground. I could see how all the unpleasant and negative energies were being drained away from the building, through the pipes into the Earth. I asked Mother Earth to transmute those energies into good ones. I saw them all going into the Earth. Then I placed the Healing and Insight reiki symbol in the building. I could see how the energy in the building was being transformed.

I was ready to go inside.

I was so insecure going into this different hospital. I didn't know where anything was and I didn't know anyone. When I found the right department, I was welcomed by a very friendly nurse. She brought me straight to Elouisa. Guess what, she had the best place again, next to the window! She is set for life, I thought, she will always have the best spot. After the excitement of her having been taken out of the incubator in the other hospital, it was a bit of a disappointment when I found her back in an incubator. Apparently the shock of transfer for these little ones is sometimes too much and makes them take a small step back. The nurse had upped the oxygen flow and Elouisa was again just in her nappy in her greenhouse. I had to let this 'step back' go. She was here, and the next step would be home.

After having been there for only ten minutes, part of the reason I was there became clear to me. A nurse came in and

The Healing of the 1lb Baby

her body language alone showed that she was an elephant in a porcelain shop. The person everybody had to listen to. She looked at me and (tried) to squash me down with just one look. The bully.

In the coming few weeks I would notice how many mothers she would upset. There were no problems with the babies. But her power of wanting to be THE one everyone had to listen to was so enormous that she would talk mean in your face. There was no hiding. Of course, having learned so much over the last months, I was not going to let her do this to me.

As her dominating energy flew towards me I (imaginarily) threw it back at her and kind of caught her in it. (It was her own energy, I didn't want it!) I put green, loving healing colour in her aura so she would learn from what she was doing.

You could see that the other nurses were used to her, but they did not like her. She would even go into dispute with the doctors.

I placed a big circle of pink light around Elouisa's incubator as protection so no outside energies could enter.

Once Elouisa was settled, she finally started being fed with bottles. She had only been fed directly into the stomach and was now ready to begin sucking by herself.

This was such an exciting moment! This process went slowly. She drank a few millilitres by herself and the rest of her feed would then be given directly into her stomach. Day by day she would start to drink more by herself.

One day I was expressing and my milk stopped. Bang. Finished, the flow stopped. First I was frustrated by this happening but then realized I had unconsciously asked for this. I really didn't want to breastfeed this time. I had done it for months/one year or more with the other three and I had had enough. I needed to stand in my own full energy without being 'sucked empty'. I had thought this and my body had reacted. The milk stopped; my wish had come true. Once my milk supply was gone from the freezer, she would receive powdered milk. This happened a few days before coming home. I had given her four months of Mummy's goodness. I felt very good having done this.

When she had been there about nine days I decided to take the children to Belgium. Here we had again the 'battle' of reactions. Nurse Bully had found a bone and couldn't let go. How dare I go on holiday while my child was in hospital! She would gossip and talk to other nurses about what kind of a mother I was to leave my child alone and so on. First, sensitive as I am, it hit me. It really, really upset me. I learned, thanks to her, to protect my own energy system so that outside comments wouldn't affect me. I imagined being surrounded by pink light. High above me, in front of me, behind me, to my sides and underneath me, I was surrounded by pink protective colour. On the outside of this 'balloon' I saw shining white light, then green and purple on the outside. I would from that day on surround myself with that light, every day. Thoughts, actions and words from other people bounce back to where they come from and stay away from you.

The reason I went to Belgium? To spend some quality time with my other children, who had missed their mum so much. It was, by the way, also the summer holidays and they have to be kept busy.

People, please, take off your blinkers!!!!

It was half way through August, and we were a good three weeks away from Elouisa being 'full term'. She was doing well. I needed a break and Andy would stay home as he needed some bonding time with his daughter Elouisa. While she had been in the other hospital, he had hardly seen her. He felt ready and was excited now she was 'bigger' to look after her and bond. He felt it was now 'safe' to bond without the risk of getting hurt.

Yes, it was hard to leave my precious baby, but it also felt good to take a breather and spend some time with the other children.

Andy kept me up to date every day with how she was doing. He sent me regular pictures. He had been able to feed her, which was lovely. She was now able to wear teeny weeny 'dolly' clothes every day. I have to admit, a few tears rolled and I couldn't wait to feed her myself.

When the end of August was approaching I was being tempted to buy loads of new stuff for Elouisa. My nesting feeling had fully hit home. Even though I still had a lot of baby stuff from Orla-Jane. I 'had' to buy everything new. I was loving this. I was finally able to tell people I had had a baby.

By the beginning of September, everything was ready. Every day for the next three weeks I would look at that empty baby basket in the lounge imagining her lying in it. Everything was pink and lovely.

The day after coming back from Belgium I went to see her. She looked so big! It had only been two weeks but she had changed so much. She looked like a baby now. A small baby, but a baby, no different from any newborn.

We had the longest cuddle ever and I gave her her bottle.

3rd of September

She had been doing so well when suddenly my happy bubble was snapped.

Andy and I arrived at the hospital when the doctor was with her. Elouisa was showing a bloated hard tummy so an infection was suspected. She had difficulty breathing and needed some more oxygen.

The doctors were suspecting necrotizing enterocolitis (NEC). This is a medical condition primarily seen in premature infants, where portions of the bowel start to die and cause an infection. It occurs post-natally and can need surgical intervention or can result in death if not noticed or treated straight away.

Elouisa was given antibiotics straight away as a precaution until more was known.

Luckily, the X-ray showed some gaseous distension only, caused by immaturity of the bowel motility.

Elouisa received another blood transfusion packed with red cells.

After three days the antibiotics were stopped as everything was fine.

After this 'event' she got stronger and stronger. She would make a right fuss when hungry and scream for England if not attended to. She was moved into a normal little bed, all snuggled up with clothes and blankets.

The hospital felt comfortable to me with all the changed energies and Nurse Bully left me alone.

20th of September

Elouisa was moved to another room. No more Intensive Care, no more Special Care, but just in a small room. She was stable on a low nasal cannula oxygen flow, which she would continue to receive at home.

She was in that room for four days before coming home. She was happy, getting fed on demand, cuddling with Mummy and receiving the last check-ups.

Her eyes and ears were confirmed fine. She had had another brain scan and the two small bleeds had seemed to dissolve.

She was still on diuretics for her oedema, which were stopped two days before coming home.

24th of September

Today was the day we had been waiting for. Today Elouisa was coming home. It felt unreal. I was extremely nervous taking her home on oxygen. The nurses kept telling me how straightforward it was but I still found this medically difficult and it scared me. What if I did something wrong or the kids turned it up or down!

Anyway, it was the way it was, she was coming home on a low flow 0.02 of oxygen via a nasal cannula and the local paediatric nursing team would in time help to wean her off. We were given an apnoea monitor, which registered her breathing. This was attached with a plaster to her tummy. It would alarm us if there was no breathing detected after a certain amount of time. I found this the best thing ever. It made sure that I slept at night and didn't constantly check on her in the daytime!

(After only three weeks, the hospital 'demanded' that monitor back as they needed it for someone else. They said I had had it long enough. I was in full panic! This little machine had made me feel at ease – what would I do now? Luckily, you can buy clip-on apnoea monitors. It is attached to the nappy and is very small. It goes up and down as the tummy moves because of the breathing. I kept it on her for several months until she started pulling it off.)

We had to wait another hour until all the last check-ups had been done. Elouisa was still swollen (oedema) around her female parts and legs.

To explain this energetically: If the swelling/water retention is around the female parts, problems here belong to a blocked Sacral chakra – energy point of emotions. Retention, not letting go, and water are metaphorically always linked to emotion. The swelling/water retention was also in her legs, and problems with the legs are related to a blockage in the Base chakra. A birth trauma has its roots in the Base chakra. She clearly had difficulty in letting go of the trauma that she had gone through and had found this emotionally very hard. The doctor had stopped her medicine against this. Once home I would treat her with Crystals.

Once it had been explained to us how to attach the nasal

cannula, how to wash her whilst on oxygen, how to change the bottle… we were ready to go.

At lunchtime, Andy and I walked out of the hospital with our fourth baby, our super strong, magical, whole love, fabulous Elouisa.

Part 3: Home

Chapter 25: Physical and Ethereal Crystal healing

We settled into a routine very quickly. I had no choice but to settle quickly. Andy had to go to work and I had to pick up the other children from pre-school and school. It was a little scary at first; everyone was looking at us, and wondering why she was on oxygen, what that big 'bottle' connected to my child was doing underneath the pushchair. I could see people stare and wonder. People looked at me with pity, wondering what illness she had.

'No, no, everyone, she is perfectly healthy!'

Some mums at the school would literally talk about her as a sick baby.

'No, no! She just needs some tiny bit of extra oxygen because of being born extremely early, not ill, SHE IS NOT ILL!'

Andy calmed me down and said, 'Does it matter what other people think?'

In the beginning, everyone would be hanging over the pram to see her, as you do, AND HOLD HER HANDS! I would cringe! I laugh about it now and I know that unless you have had a baby in Intensive Care, you have no idea how manically crazy you act when it comes to hygiene.

I simply started telling people straight away, 'Please understand that we have just come out of a hospital where hand gel and soaps are used constantly. Give her time to adjust to the not washed hands world, please.'

My close friends would remember and have respect for that and even tell their kids off when they had their little hands all over Elouisa.

People would simply not understand the seriousness of hand washing and the worry, as a mother, concerning hygiene. When you have been in a hospital environment for so long and when you have seen what your child has been through, you understand. That was very clear.

After a few weeks of frustrating incidents, I would leave a bottle of hand gel at the front door and anyone coming in had to use it. You know what – Elouisa was my baby, I had the right to ask that and if someone didn't understand, that was their problem.

Once home I could finally heal with Crystals. She was still so small and didn't move around much so I put Crystals in her socks on the undersides of her feet. I have to say that I always kept a close eye on her and took them out for the night! Always keep an eye on children when using Crystals on them and make sure it is safe!!!

My confidence was growing, I was no longer 'embarrassed' for the healing work I was doing. I used to not talk about it with anyone. I didn't want people to think I was weird or mad. Having Elouisa had given me an enormous confidence boost. I did not have to hide what I did and who I was any longer. The Universe knew exactly why they had sent me Elouisa.

As I already said, every chakra gives energy into the body and therefore influences the organs and their functions, blood circulation, hormones, emotions and thoughts.

That's why it is so vitally important that there are no blockages and the energy can flow beautifully so we have no physical, emotional or psychological problems and we simply live happily and healthily.

The human tissue exists out of energy vibrations. Crystals also have energy vibrations.

When there are blockages, pain or disease, the vibration of wherever the problem is has changed. By wearing a Crystal, its vibration will influence the changed frequencies in the body and bring it back into balance. The body will react to the vibration of the stone.

Crystals also have an incredible influence on emotional and psychological health.

It is hugely important to find the right stone, or combination of several stones.

When healing a physical problem, also find a Crystal that heals the chakra where the energy has stopped flowing and is causing the problem, so the root is pulled out. Otherwise the problem might be back in no time. So choose a stone for the problem AND the related chakra.

I used the following Crystals for healing on Elouisa:
- Sodalite: Sodalite gives enormous peace and helps against water retention. This way the water retention could be healed and she would feel at peace and relaxed. The water retention reduced very quickly and healed in no time. Elouisa was the most relaxed and happy baby I've ever known. Sodalite is a crystal that heals the Third Eye. In the Third Eye lie problems with brain, eyes… Healing with this stone would make sure her Third Eye was beautifully cleansed.
- Tiger Eye: Tiger Eye is an incredible healer for lungs and airways. Because the medical world had stuck the tag 'chronic lung disease' on her as a 'result' of her extremely premature birth, her lungs needed

strengthening. Tiger Eye also protects against negative energies. Tiger Eye is a Crystal that heals in particular the Sacral chakra, the energy point of emotions (which was in need of healing after her emotional roller coaster birth and hospital stay) and the Solar Plexus, the energy point of the will. Via family circles (explained earlier), she could easily have taken over my guilt and shame, which could block her Solar Plexus. Uncertain situations – as the first four months of her life were – caused by the possibility of having a blocked Solar Plexus. Suppression of the will – as she was only able to lie there and 'undergo' – is also a big cause of the Solar Plexus getting blocked. As a result, many (extremely) prematurely born babies suffer from reflux. Reflux is one of the physical problems that can occur when having a blocked Solar Plexus. Elouisa had no problems at all with reflux! A good working Solar Plexus would also help her to have no muscular problems (see Chapter 6). Again, many prem babies have weak muscles and there lies the root energetically. Elouisa never had weak muscles or problems with muscles.

- Chalcedony: Chalcedony strengthens the bond between mother and child, which I thought was helpful seeing that she had missed sixteen weeks in the womb. Chalcedony heals traumas so was perfect to heal Elouisa's birth trauma. Chalcedony is a healer of all emotions. What she had been through was very emotional for her; the bloated tummy, water retention around the female parts had already physically shown that there was a blockage. Chalcedony would restore the energy vibrations and make sure there were no emotional blockages left. Chalcedony heals in particular the Throat chakra. Being born that early and being pushed, prodded and handled whenever needed, can have a devastating effect on the person in communication. She wasn't able to say what she was feeling, she wasn't able to 'defend' herself; she just had to undergo it. This could have blocked her Throat chakra, the energy point of communication. Many children born extremely prematurely end up with problems in swallowing, and the roots of that problem lie exactly there. So Chalcedony would also help to make sure that the energy in her Throat chakra was flowing nicely and she would not have any problems with swallowing.

Every time the health visitor or nurse came to check on her progress, they asked if she had any stones in her socks. It was nice how respectful they were towards my healing techniques with Elouisa. At the end of the day, they could see how well Elouisa was doing...

Chapter 26: Eating

It is 'typical' for (extremely) premature babies to have eating problems.

Eating problems – as seen in Chapter 6 – have their seat in the Base chakra, the Solar Plexus and Heart chakra.

To sum it all up: A premature baby undergoes:
- Long treatment by doctors/hospitals, sometimes surgery (Base chakra)
- Birth trauma (Base chakra)
- Shame/taken over from parents (Solar Plexus)
- Guilt/taken over from parents (Solar Plexus)
- Uncertain situations (Solar Plexus)
- Suppression of the will (Solar Plexus)
- Missing out on a lot of body contact/physical feeling of love from the mother because of lying in an incubator (Heart chakra)

On top of that, the child is not able to communicate and gets a blocked Throat chakra, which can give problems with swallowing.

As a result, the perfect cocktail can be created for digestive, eating and swallowing problems.

Elouisa had none of these.

On the advice of the paediatric nurse I introduced solids when Elouisa was seven months/corrected age four months. When it comes to weaning, this is the only time where you don't look at the corrected age. A premature baby needs to start going on solids at the age of between five and eight months (counted from birth). However, it is best to wait until they are at least three months corrected age so that they will have developed sufficient head control.

It is best to start at that age; otherwise you might miss a good time for your baby to develop eating skills. At that age, babies are usually willing to try new flavours but as they grow older they can become more reluctant.

Elouisa looked extremely small in that big eating chair but I trusted and followed the nurse's advice.

It did happen a few times that Elouisa suddenly shut her throat and started choking. Luckily I had followed first aid before leaving the hospital. I would have to tip her tummy and face downwards and tap firmly between the shoulder blades. The food would than fall out and only left us in a bit of a shock.

After several weeks I started realizing that infections only pop up when the emotional stress becomes too high… which would than block the Sacral chakra and result in infections or other physical pains. I knew Elouisa was happy and content and was energetically being healed with the Crystals. When that realization came, I started going to the supermarkets and shops again. I had tried to avoid those places as they are packed with germs through the air conditioning system. From than on, I would take her everywhere. I would, before I left, imagine her in a big pink balloon that nothing could penetrate. Everything would bounce off that protective balloon and she would stay in her strength.

A few weeks before Elouisa turned one year, she was weaned off the oxygen. We could clearly see that she had enough as she kept pulling off the tube. This weaning happened very gradually over the course of several weeks. A few hours off, then monitor the amount of oxygen in her blood and then on the oxygen again. When all was well the hours off would be increased. This went very smoothly with Elouisa.

The 16th of May she was released off the extra oxygen! What a happy day!!! No more restriction around the house, no more tripping over the wire or worrying that the other kids might fiddle with it. We could just pick her up and move around freely!

The 1st of July, against all well meant advice from the doctors, Elouisa went to nursery. I knew she would be fine. Elouisa was a normal child. Her traumas and all problems linked to her extremely premature birth had been healed. When it is healed, it is gone. The roots were pulled out, it was gone and so had no more influence on her! She absolutely loved nursery and had no more colds or coughs than the other full term born friends.

If sniffles or coughs appeared, I would from now on place Ethereal Crystals.

I had physical crystals all over the house, on window sills and on the terrace. I used them when working on clients. One day I stood there thinking out loud how actually all the Crystal cleansing and charging was a lot of work and very time consuming. I loved working with them but I had enough of all the 'looking after'. I didn't have to wait long for the Universe to give me an answer/solution.

I was conducting healing on a client. I gave a specific Crystal to my client to hold while I was working on that specific chakra to help the healing along. The client kept the Crystals in her hands even when the next one was added.

I felt that this lady needed these Crystals with her for longer but that was not possible when the session was finished. As I was thinking this, my spirit guides told me to 'imagine'/place the Crystal into the chakra of my client so it could keep working on her healing when she went home. So I did. It felt very strong and had an incredible healing power as I placed the 'imagined stones' in her chakras.

A few days later, I was on the phone with my friend Carine, who started telling me about Ethereal Crystals! I had never heard of them before and the link to the healing I did a few days before was made immediately. I was, of course, ecstatic when she told me that the healing I had conducted has a name!!! She then sent me the attunements and information behind the Ethereal Crystals. I have worked with them ever since.

When we work with Ethereal Crystals, the Universe directly gives us the strength/power of the Crystal, which we then place simply by intention. The strength of Ethereal Crystals is about four hundred times stronger than those found on Earth, because they are pure and come directly from another dimension.

It is possible to capture these energies purely by intention.

I love working with Ethereal Crystals and always do in my practice.

- The healing energy is always in its full form and strength.
- You don't need to look after the stone.
- The stone is always 'the right one' for you, in contrast to a physical Crystal where you have to find the stone that works for you.
- You can use Ethereal Crystals even if you are at the other side of the world and want to give healing and protection or give energy to someone.
- Once the energy of the stone is placed it fades away by itself when it is no longer needed. Unlike material Crystals they cannot be dislodged by movement or

> activity. You can place them in or on everything and everyone simply by positive strong intention.
> - You can make gem elixirs in seconds.
> - You can also strengthen a material stone by using the strength of your ability to work with Ethereal Crystals.

I still have Crystals lying around but have fully diverted to healing with Ethereal Crystals. More about this can be found in my book *Heal by Intention – Crystal Learning and Oracle Cards.*

When Elouisa had the sniffles I would place an Ethereal Crystal Agate in her nasal cavity, Aquamarine on her Throat chakra. They would heal the cold very quickly.

For a cough: Tiger Eye on the bronchi; Tiger Eye on the Solar Plexus; Amber in the lungs; Chalcedony on the airways; Chrysocolla on her Heart chakra and Aquamarine on her Throat chakra. I would confirm via her Higher Self that our natural state is perfect health. It would always pass quite quickly.

Elouisa had to go back to the hospital for her ears to be checked. The doctor had told me they were fine but wanted a closer monitoring because she had found fluid in her right middle ear. The cause might have been a cold but I didn't want to take any risks.

I wanted to heal before going back for the check-up. I was going to place Crystals but felt that psychic surgery was needed. Of course, to be able to do that I wanted to know what an ear looked like on the inside. The week before the check-up we were at the Science Museum with the boys and guess what looked me straight in the eye: The inside of an ear! (The Universe always answers your questions). I had a good look and made a photograph with my mind.

Once home I said Elouisa's name out loud and pictured the inside of her ear. I imagined a small pipette going into her middle ear to retract all the fluid. Once all the fluid was gone, I placed the reiki healing symbol and an Ethereal Crystal blue Agate in her middle ear. At the check-up it was confirmed that her ears were clear and healthy.

Elouisa started walking at 22 months/corrected age 18 months – no different from full term born children.

After we came home from the four month two day hospital stay, Elouisa received the best after-care ever from specialist doctors, nurses and health visitors, physiotherapists, occupational therapists, nutritionists and so on.

Elouisa's nickname with them was 'Miracle Baby'. Everyone knew who they were talking about when they said 'Miracle Baby'.

The statistics in the UK say the following:
Babies born early may not survive, may survive and be healthy or may survive but have long-term problems and disabilities. The chance of survival increases with each additional week of pregnancy and the risk of disability reduces.
Born at 24 weeks, 4–5 in 10 survive, of whom half have moderate to severe disabilities.
Elouisa belongs to the very small percentage of 2 in 10 babies who come out perfectly.
Is it luck, is it life, is it meant to be? I believe it was the strong collaboration of medical and spiritual healing. Times change and the awareness of humans grows.
The mind is so incredibly strong! The Universe knows only love, health and happiness, and we are a part of that!
We are from nature perfectly healthy. We must let go of past hang-ups via psychic surgery, physical and Ethereal Crystals, help from Celestial beings, past life regression... and know that we are all one. Perfect health, whole love and full happiness THAT, is what we are.

Believe in miracles.